First Line Guide Psychiatric and Behavioral Medicine

Mike Sacks, DMSc, PA-C
Rebecca DePalma, DMSc, PA-C

Contributing Editors:

Talya Cohen, PsyD
Bracha Stern, PsyD
Hayley Knostman, DMSc, PA-C, CAQ-Psy
Stephanie O'Malley, M.S., PA-C, CAQ-Psy

Published By First Line Guide, LLC June 2024

First Line Guide Psychiatric and Behavioral Medicine

ISBN # 9798986546919

Cover & Chapter Art: ID 96544167 © Hendraxaverius | Dreamstime.com

MEET THE AUTHORS

Mike Sacks, DMSc, PA-C

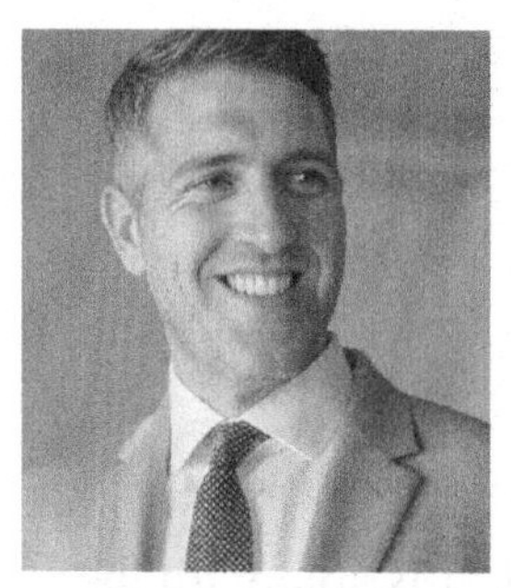

Mike Sacks is a family medicine and emergency medicine PA from Brooklyn, NY, living and practicing in Westchester County, a suburb of New York City. After studying emergency management as an undergraduate, he studied PA medicine at the Hofstra University PA program and later earned his Doctorate of Medical Science from the University of Lynchburg. Mike is a PA educator, serving as an adjunct professor and clinical preceptor for multiple local PA programs and has lectured on a variety of medical topics at several PA conferences and for more than forty PA programs throughout the United States. In November 2021, Mike was recognized by the AAPA for his role as a clinical preceptor and awarded the CPAAPA credential for his dedication to training future PAs.

Outside of clinical practice and education, Mike serves as a consulting editor for a major peer-reviewed medical journal and is a member of several local medical task forces and committees.

ACKNOWLEDGEMENTS

There are several people to whom I owe an enormous debt of gratitude for the role they played in bringing the First Line Guide series to fruition.

First, I would like to thank my wife, Joanna. Like everything else I've done professionally, it would have been impossible to write this book without your steadfast support. Thank you for always offering me the flexibility and leeway to pursue my goals.

To my children, Samara and Ari, I am sorry for having missed so many evenings and weekends with you as I wrote this book. I'm so incredibly excited to make up for that lost time in the weeks and months ahead. I love you both to an extent you will not understand until you have children of your own.

To my brother Joe, I am grateful for all the contributions you have made to this project that so many will never know about.

To my co-authors, editors and to the many contributors, to not just this book but to content in the FLG catalog, past present and future – my most sincere thanks. First Line Guide has, and will continue to be a community work with contributions from so many, without whom this wouldn't be the same.

Rebecca DePalma, DMSc, PA-C

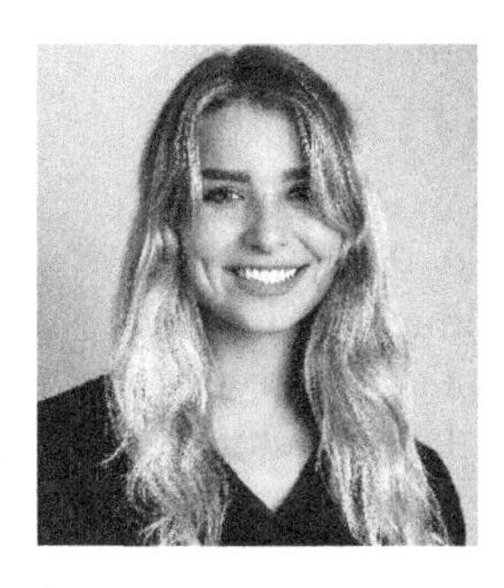

Rebecca is a practicing psychiatry PA, originally from the Seattle area of Washington. She received her Bachelor of Science from Loyola Marymount University in Los Angeles, where she graduated with honors as magna cum laude. She then went to PA school at Pacific University, earning her master's degree in PA studies. Thereafter, she earned her Doctorate of Medical Science. In addition to her clinical work as a psychiatry PA, Rebecca is a preceptor and mentor for future providers, guest professor at several universities, and author. She is dedicated to guiding students and advancing the PA profession.

ACKNOWLEDGEMENTS

I am very thankful for the path that led me to where I am today. The experiences I have garnered and the people I have met along the way have made my journey an absolute joy that I will always cherish.

To my parents, Vince and Patricia, brother and sister, Joseph and Victoria, and grandmother Renate for their unwavering belief in me. Your love and support have never faltered no matter the venture I dedicate myself to. And to my friends across the country, including Nina, for continually cheering me on and believing in any and all crazy endeavors that I put my mind to.

From preceptor to co-author, Mike, thank you for your supreme trust and belief in me. I am forever thankful I took the plunge as a PA student to set off for a rotation across the country, to our pursuits to assist future and current medical providers, striving to augment the profession – and this is only the beginning.

CONTRIBUTING EDITORS

Stephanie O'Malley, M.S., PA-C, CAQ-Psy

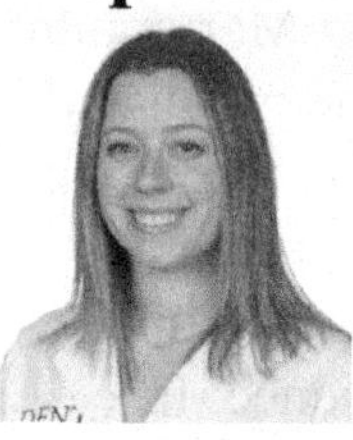

Stephanie is a psychiatric PA working in Buffalo, NY, and a graduate of the Daemen University PA Program. Stephanie works in a busy outpatient clinic which offers both traditional medication management and interventional psychiatry treatments. To optimize available treatment modalities to her patients, Stephanie is also in the process of gathering clinical research to support the implementation of botulinum toxin for the treatment of depression. In addition to her clinical work in outpatient psychiatry, she has provided mentorship and has been a preceptor for PA students from several local universities. Stephanie strives to promote mental health through lifestyle including dietary and exercise interventions in addition to medication management.

Hayley Knostman, DMSc, PA-C, CAQ-Psy

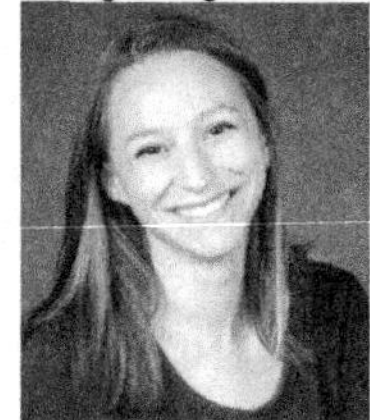

Hayley is a psychiatric PA from Dayton, Ohio, living and practicing in Durham, North Carolina, at an eating disorder specialty hospital. She is a graduate of the Pennsylvania State University College of Medicine PA program. She was a National Health Service Corps Scholar, and completed her service in Yakima, Washington, working at a community mental health center and FQHC. She has since earned a CAQ in Psychiatry, and her DMSc with a concentration in Psychiatry from Rocky Mountain University of Health Professions. Hayley precepts students and enjoys having future PA students shadow her in practice. She serves as the Triangle Area regional chapter president of the North Carolina Academy of Physician Assistants.

Talya Cohen, PsyD

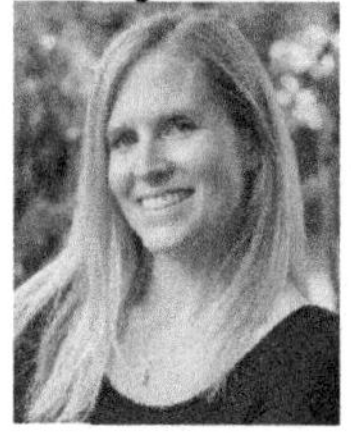

Talya is a clinical psychologist licensed in New York and Connecticut, and the co-founder of Impact Psychological Services, a large, evidence-based, integrative mental health care practice servicing Westchester County, NY. Talya works with adults, adolescents, children, and families struggling with a variety of emotional, behavioral, and relational challenges. Talya utilizes an integrated therapeutic approach to treat the specific needs of the individuals she works with - incorporating psychodynamic, cognitive behavioral, family systems, and mindfulness interventions. Talya helps clients improve and repair relationships, process painful experiences, alleviate stress and anxiety, identify and challenge maladaptive thoughts and behaviors and ultimately find the inner strength to live their best lives.

HOW TO GET INVOLVED

This book is the product of a collaborative effort of clinicians across the mental health and wellness space. We are grateful to all those who made contributions, and we will be forever grateful to those who continue to make contributions moving forward as medicine and our understanding of mental health in continually evolving. We invite all readers to play a role by submitting corrections, changes, recommendations, thoughts, and ideas.

To contribute, email info@firstlineguide.com, and be sure to identify the disease or subject in question, your edits, the page number, and any citations.

You can also contact us on Instagram:
Rebecca DePalma @rebeccawestcoastpa
Mike Sacks @family_med_pa
First Line Guide @firstlineguide

TABLE OF CONTENTS

Psychiatry Clerkship

Rotations can be intimidating, especially when rotating in a specialty. You will encounter things you have never learned –this is a great thing, and why rotations are such a beautiful learning experience. Embrace the opportunity to learn more in-depth on topics where previously you may have just scratched the surface.

This advice can be adapted for any rotation. Always attentively listen to your preceptor, and see how they wish to integrate you into the patient process. If you don't know something or need clarification, don't be afraid to speak up and ask for help! No one will expect you to know everything. In fact, they probably expect you to know little to nothing, as each is assumed to be the first rotation of its kind for every student that walks through the door. Take notes and be inquisitive, compiling questions to set aside for later. See if they would prefer you to ask questions throughout the day or to save them for all together at the end of the day. Pay attention to details so you can learn something the first time you are shown and try your best to not repeat the same mistake twice. Try to get to know your preceptor(s) in addition to other workers, be personable and write down names. Recognize that while this is a clinical rotation to you, you are really an observer in the lives of all that work there and as such should show the gratitude that warrants. Be professional, respectful, and authentic to yourself. Above all, believe in yourself and you will do well!

What to Expect

Psychiatry rotations can vary vastly depending on the types of facilities – some are inpatient, some are outpatient, with v51arying levels of acuity. Some will utilize telepsychiatry and others will be in person. Some may also have separate therapists for a counseling component in addition to the medical side of psychiatry.

For psychiatry, you can expect the diagnosis, treatment, and monitoring of conditions such as:

- Anxiety
- Depression
- Bipolar disorder
- Schizophrenia
- Insomnia
- Substance abuse
- and much more -see sections 2-10.

If severe, inpatient treatment may be necessary. You will become adept with the medication management of these conditions amongst comorbid disease states, including lab monitoring and appropriate referrals.

Inpatient – Patients are admitted either within a traditional hospital setting, or one dedicated to psychiatric care. This service is generally reserved for patients that need to be monitored closely and regularly as they would not be safe in an outpatient setting.

Outpatient – Patients receive medical care or treatment without hospital admission, typically in a clinic setting. Outpatient care management is well suited for stable patients that are not considered to be an immediate risk to themselves or others, and do not require close monitoring.

New Grad Advice

If you are a new grad starting in psychiatry, it will likely be overwhelming at first. Not only are you in a specialty, but will likely be using some intense medications, with patients at times in particularly precarious situations and mental states. This can be stressful but will become easier with time. We recommend having a comprehensive list of all the medications you will be using and the "need-to-know" aspects of those medications such as starting doses, side effects, if lab follow-up is required, and common interactions to watch for.

When it comes to controlled substances, set rules hard and fast for patients on what your policies are. Examples such as – requiring records from a previously diagnosing provider prior to taking over a medication regimen, requiring a urine drug screen before prescribing medications known for abuse potential, etc., and remember you are not obligated to take over an already established medication regimen if it is something you would not have done yourself. You and the patient must mutually agree on a treatment plan that is best for their overall collective mental and physical health.

As you progress, you will quickly learn your favorite medications and what works best for differing disease states with varying constellations of symptoms.

Differential Diagnoses

As we go through the various psychiatric diagnoses in this text, we want to add a notice that this is not all encompassing of all diagnoses that can contribute to psychiatric complaints and disorders.

Psychiatry is an ever-evolving field, that needs more research, and more is constantly being learned. We want to take a moment to point out the many diseases of other specialties that can have psychiatric intersection. When someone comes to you with psychiatric complaints, be sure to not close your mind off to an expanded differential.

Ex. B12 deficiency, Cushing's disease, PCOS, thyroid diseases, autoimmune encephalitis, infections, dementia, other CNS diseases/tumors, and even diagnoses as simple as a UTI can cause psychiatric symptoms. This list could go on, so for all psych-related symptoms be sure to be thorough in your assessment and consider all possibilities outside beyond the realm of psychiatry.

Clinical Pearls

- Low dose second generation antipsychotics (i.e., aripiprazole, risperidone) are used by some as an off label adjunctive therapy to SSRIs to treat severe depression, ruminations, and anxious distress.

- Buspirone and bupropion are both used off-label to treat sexual side effects associated with SSRIs.

- While anxiety and depressive disorders are frequent in patients with ADHD, symptoms of the three conditions overlap. In patients newly presenting with concerns for ADHD, treating their mood first can aid in ruling ADHD in or out.

- Low dose lithium has demonstrated efficacy in treating "impulsive-aggressive" behavior which when used in patients with suicidal ideation is believed to lower the likelihood of suicidal behavior (Benard, et al. 2016)

- Changing psychiatric medications due to pregnancy should be given great consideration before any decision is made. The benefits of stable mental health may often outweigh the risks associated with most non-teratogenic medications. Defer to patient's OBGYN when needed.

- Consider bipolar spectrum disorders in patients with depression presenting with attention difficulties, anhedonia, agitation, and anger (the four A's). In all patients with psychiatric complaints, screen for any history of mania

- After two weeks of treatment with SSRI/SNRI patients should be reassessed. Those that report "zero-response" (<20% improvement) at this time are likely to experience minimal further benefit and a change of medication or addition of an adjunctive medication could be considered (Hicks, et al. 2019). However, some patients will still have benefit when medication is on for full 6-8 weeks, some may also need a dose increase/adjustment.

- Patient's presenting with diagnoses made by others should be considered for re-evaluation as treating based on someone else's potentially incorrect diagnosis benefits neither the provider nor the patient.

- Regularly administering medications achieves a given steady-state concentration after approximately 4 to 5 half-lives without any further accumulation in the body with repeated doses. By calculating the time it takes to reach 4-5 half-lives, you can establish the ideal time to measure drug levels to assess efficacy.

- Establish realistic expectations with regard to how long it will take for patients to notice benefit to a given medication. Patients that are not expecting a rapid response are more likely to be compliant long enough to appreciate a benefit.

- When making a choice between multiple medication options consider the benefits a side-effect profile might offer. For example, patients with depression that are having trouble sleeping, and loss of appetite may find all three symptoms improved with mirtazapine. Or patients with depression and coexisting low energy may benefit from bupropion.

- Be thorough. No matter the chief complaint, make sure you are also screening for anxiety, depression, substance use, and suicidal ideation.

- Consider alcohol or drug use as a cause in all new-onset psychosis.

- Safety plans are an evidence-based and effective technique to reduce suicide risk. Documentation of a safety plan is also protective of the provider. For example, the clinician can ask: "What will you do if it is 2:00am and you are thinking of killing yourself?" and then help the patient plan out coping strategies and write them down. Sample solutions may include: "I will call my aunt, or listen to music, or write in my journal, or exercise, or watch a TV series." (AAP, 2023)

- Don't be afraid of uncomfortable silence from a patient. Sometimes waiting longer allows them to collect their thoughts or say something more that they would have otherwise withheld.

- With early treatment, a majority of those that experience first-episode psychosis will achieve full remission.

- To build report and increase patient comfort, identify topics your patient enjoys and them bring up during each visit, as encounters can become deeply personal and emotionally challenging.

- Most adolescents who think about suicide or engage in non-suicidal self-harm will not make an attempt on their life (Mars, et al. 2019).

However, those that have previously attempted suicide should be viewed as the most likely to make future attempts.

- In pediatric populations where custody is shared between divorced or separated parents obtain consent from both parents before starting medications.
- Be mindful of the whole patient and other chronic conditions they may have. Many psychiatric medications can impact other medical conditions, so be attentive to how those interact and involve other specialists as needed.
- Obtain a detailed family history. Many psychiatric conditions are known to have strong hereditary/genetic factors.

- Nutrition, sleep, exercise, and other lifestyle interventions should be viewed as an important part of any mental health treatment plan.

- Be aware of the lethal doses of all medications you prescribe and when there is any concern of suicidal ideation, provide fewer pills than necessary for an intentional overdose.

- Take the extra time to educate your patients on their condition, and the treatments you are providing. Informed patients are far more compliant than those that feel they are blindly trusting your judgement.

- Help end the stigma associated with psychiatric conditions. By perpetuating the normalcy of mental health struggles, you empower your patients to accept treatment they may otherwise have not.

- Be empathetic. Regardless of the field of medicine you work in, we often encounter patients on some of the worst days of their lives. An empathetic encounter can be lifesaving for some patients.

PHARMACOLOGY

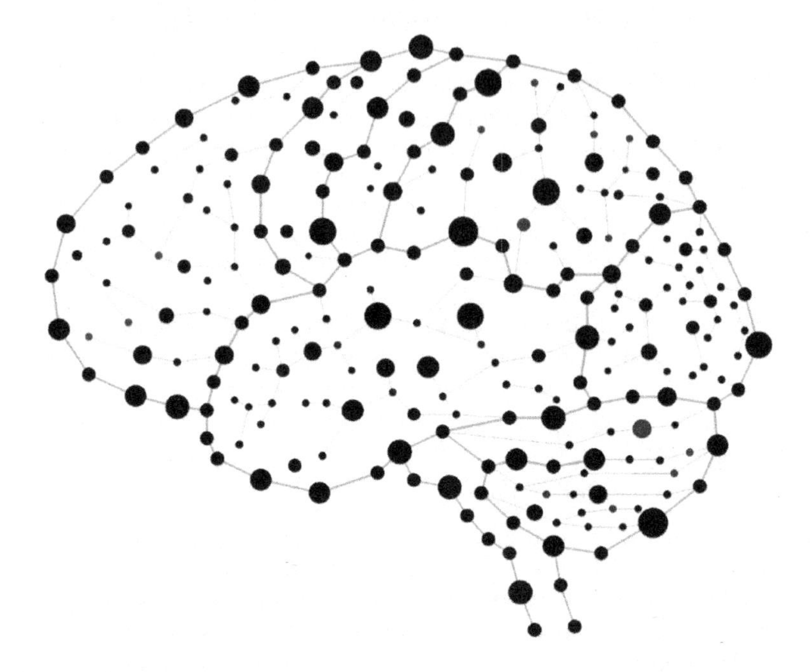

Throughout this text, medication class names are referenced such as "antipsychotics" or "antidepressants". It is important to note these treat more than their listed name. For example: "antipsychotics" are often used to augment more traditional medications in treatment-resistant depression or obsessive-compulsive disorder, in addition to their traditional use in psychotic disorders. These can also be conceptualized based on their mechanisms of action, such as dopaminergic antagonists, or dopaminergic-serotonergic agents. Likewise, antidepressants are used for a multitude of conditions beyond depression. It is important to acknowledge that some traditional medication class names such as antipsychotics, or even antidepressants for those that do not have depression, may be viewed as off-putting or with a negative connotation by some patient populations. Therefore, it is crucial to educate patients to rectify these common misunderstandings, which can also promote better compliance.

Neurotransmitters

An imbalance in neurotransmitters can be both genetic and environmental.

Excitatory

- **Dopamine:** motivation, pleasure, desire, movement, learning; (can also be inhibitory)
- **Norepinephrine:** energy, alertness, concentration
- **Glutamate:** cognition, memory, creation of neural connections

Inhibitory

- **Serotonin:** mood, emotional state, attention, thought processing, sleep, appetite, digestion, urge control, memory
- **GABA:** calmness, clarity, focus, motor control, vision

Genetics

Genetic testing is frequently used in psychiatry to both isolate genetic predisposition to disease, as well as one's ability to metabolize medication effectively.

- **MTHFR Gene Mutation**– MTHFR is an enzyme required to convert folic acid into an active form called L-methylfolate that is used in the production of mood regulating neurotransmitters such as serotonin, dopamine, and norepinephrine. Those with this mutation have may not adequately produce these neurotransmitters and thus experience treatment failure SSRIs and SNRIs. The MTHFR gene mutations can be identified with genetic screening.
  - **Treatment:** L-methyl folate as monotherapy or added to SSRI
- **Pharmacogenomic testing** – Ninety-five percent of the population are estimated to carry at least one genetic variant that interferes with their ability to metabolize at least one medication. Pharmacogenomic testing is used to identify patients with genetic variants that put them at risk of adverse drug reactions and sub-optimal therapy. In the United States (US), an estimated 5% to 10% of patients are poor metabolizers of CYP2D6 which would impact their ability to metabolize medications like Fluoxetine, Paroxetine, and aripiprazole. An estimated 2% to 15% of those in the US are poor metabolizers of CYP2C19, which would impact their metabolization of medications like citalopram, escitalopram, and sertraline. When patients repeatedly fail treatments, many providers find use of pharmacogenomic testing to identify medications more likely to be effective. (David, et al. 2021, Pyzocha 2021)

Psychiatric Treatment Options

For all psychiatric/mood disorders, using a multifactorial approach is important. This means combining both ***psychotherapy*** *and* ***medication*** *along with* ***lifestyle changes*** *and habit formations together for* ***the most successful outcomes****.*

Lifestyle: Nutrition, exercise, coping skills, positive relationships, living environment, activities that foster a positive mood, work, patient goals

Anti-depressants/Anti-anxiety

Selective Serotonin Reuptake Inhibitors (SSRI)

- **First line therapy for depression and anxiety**
  - *Note – treatment for depression and anxiety often overlap*
    - Essential to rule out bipolar disorder (can trigger mania)
  - May take **1-2 months to reach therapeutic effect**
    - Patients are often under the impression that starting an SSRI means they'll be on one indefinitely. Clarifying that treatment is generally 6-18 months may assuage some concerns. Select patients are better managed staying on an SSRI and may elect to stay on longer, but many are able to discontinue the medication after a prolonged period of improvement.
  - MOA: Selectively block presynaptic reuptake of serotonin → Increase serotonin CNS activity
- Fluoxetine (Prozac)
  - Approved in children over age 8**; longest half-life** so lowest risk of SSRI discontinuation syndrome
    - Available in liquid formulation for those that are tablet averse
    - Long half-life → good choice for patients with poor compliance
    - Typically taken in the morning
    - One of the lower risks of weight gain
    - Available in weekly formulation
  - FDA approved for MDD, OCD, Bulimia nervosa, Panic disorder, Bipolar depression (adjunct), treatment-resistant depression; used off-label for social anxiety disorder, PTSD
- Sertraline (Zoloft)
  - Approved in children over age 8; serotonergic and histaminergic

- Lower risk in breastfeeding and pregnancy when compared to other SSRIs
    - Good option in women of child baring age
    - Available in liquid formulation
    - Typically taken in the evening/at night (due to histaminergic action)
- Known for diarrhea as an early side effect (squirt-raline)
- FDA approved for MDD, OCD, Panic disorder, PTSD, Premenstrual dysphoric disorder, social anxiety; used off-label for GAD, separation anxiety disorder

- Paroxetine (Paxil)
    - MOST associated with **weight gain** and **cardiac abnormalities**; sexual dysfx common
    - Sometimes used for patients with need for weight gain
    - FDA approved for MDD, OCD, Panic disorder, social anxiety disorder, PTSD, GAD, PMDD
    - Potent CYP450 2D6 inhibitor

- Fluvoxamine (Luvox)
    - Commonly used for treating OCD
    - Long half-life, forgiving with missed doses and low incidence of withdrawal with discontinuation
    - FDA approved for MDD, OCD, Bulimia nervosa, Panic disorder, Bipolar depression (adjunct), treatment-resistant depression; used off-label for social anxiety disorder, PTSD

- Citalopram (Celexa)
    - Interacts with many other medications, including some antibiotics and NSAIDS
    - QT prolongation

FDA approved for MDD; used off-label for OCD, GAD, PTSD, PMDD, social anxiety, panic disorder

- Escitalopram (Lexapro)
    - QT prolongation
    - Anecdotally avoided in patients with migraine history due to risk of triggering
    - FDA approved for MDD, GAD; used off-label for OCD, PTSD, PMDD, social anxiety, panic disorder

Common class adverse effects

- **GI disturbances**
- **Sexual dysfunction** (decreased libido / anorgasmia),
- Sleep disturbances

Other class adverse events

- Headache, tremor, weight gain, suicide risk, **mania/hypomania** (for those with underlying/undiagnosed bipolar disorder), QT prolongation, hyponatremia, **serotonin syndrome**, antiplatelet effects, SIADH
  - *Although similar side effect profiles are possible within the class, clinically a patient may experience a particular side effect on one SSRI that they may or may not have the same issues with on an alternative SSRI, but this varies for each individual patient.*
- **Black box warning**: increased **suicidality** in **children/adolescents/young adults** (<25 y.o.)

Serotonin Syndrome

- Vague constellation of symptoms secondary to excessive serotonin accumulation
  - Rare; Patients who are on SSRIs or other psychotropic medications (typically high doses and multiple agents). Other medications that increase risk include cough suppressants (such as Dextromethorphan), or abortive migraine medication (such as Sumatriptan). There are many other classes of medications that can also increase the risk.
- Symptoms
  - Triad of **AMS, autonomic instability, and neuromuscular abnormality**
  - Autonomic → Diaphoresis, shivering, tachycardia, hyperthermia, BP/HR swings
  - CNS → Agitation, hallucinations, seizure, coma, dizziness, ataxia
  - GI → Nausea, vomiting, diarrhea
  - Neuromuscular → Weakness, hyperreflexia, muscle rigidity/myoclonus, incoordination, tremors
- Treatment
  - **Cyproheptadine** (5HT-2 antagonist)
  - Decrease/lower provoking agent(s)

SSRI Discontinuation Syndrome

- Occurs with **abrupt withdrawal of antidepressants that were taken for at least 6 weeks**
  - Can be avoided with a slow taper off of medication
  - Most likely to happen with **paroxetine** and **sertraline**, due to their shorter half-lives
  - Least likely to happen with fluoxetine (Prozac) due to its long half-life
- Symptoms

    - **FINISH** (flu-like symptoms, insomnia, nausea, imbalance, sensory disturbances, hyperarousal)
- Educate patients not to abruptly stop taking their medications and **prescribe a taper** to minimize discontinuation symptoms (can taper quicker if doses are low)
    - May also swap to fluoxetine to aid with taper down due to long half-life
- Can prescribe a cross-taper if swapping to an alternative SSRI, where you wean one off while starting the alternative. Follow cross-tapering instructions per each individual rx.

Anxiolytic

- Buspirone (Buspar)
    - MOA: serotonin partial agonist
    - Indicated for anxiety

Selective Serotonin-Norepinephrine Reuptake Inhibitors (SNRI)

- Often 2nd line after failing SSRIs, would replace the SSRI
    - MOA: **Inhibit the reuptake of serotonin, norepinephrine, and dopamine reuptake**
    - Indicated for depression and anxiety, first line agents in patients with significant fatigue or pain syndromes in association with depression

- Venlafaxine (Effexor)
    - Requires good patient compliance
    - Avoid abrupt discontinuation due to withdrawal sx, requires longer taper off
        - *Pearl – adding fluoxetine (Prozac) can make the wean off of Effexor easier, due to fluoxetine's long half-life*
    - FDA approved for depression, GAD, social anxiety, panic disorder, separation anxiety; used off-label for PTSD, PMDD

- Desvenlafaxine (Pristique)
    - Active metabolite of venlafaxine
    - Known for significant withdrawal symptoms with rapid discontinuation
    - Dose-dependent increase in blood pressure
    - FDA approved for MDD; used off-label for GAD, social anxiety, panic disorder, PTSD, PMDD, vasomotor symptoms, fibromyalgia

- Duloxetine (Cymbalta)
    - Commonly used for chronic pain (low back pain, osteoarthritis, and fibromyalgia)

- "Depression *hurts*, Cymbalta helps" was the original ad campaign which makes it easy to remember it's pain indication.
- Contraindicated in patients with hepatic insufficiency
- Not recommended for use in patients with alcohol use disorder
- FDA approved for MDD, GAD, chronic musculoskeletal pain, fibromyalgia, diabetic peripheral neuropathic pain; used off-label for other anxiety disorders, other neuropathic pain, chronic pain

- Desvenlafaxine (Pristiq)
  - Active metabolite of venlafaxine
  - Known for significant withdrawal symptoms with rapid discontinuation
  - Dose-dependent increase in blood pressure
  - More potent 5HT reuptake inhibition than NE, but greater action at NE than venlafaxine
  - FDA approved for MDD; used off-label for GAD, social anxiety, panic disorder, PTSD, PMDD, vasomotor symptoms, fibromyalgia

- Levomilnacipran (Fetzima)
  - Renally excreted, dose adjustments indicated for patients with renal impairment
  - Greater NE reuptake inhibition than other SNRIs – unclear clinical significance
  - FDA approved for MDD; used off-label for fibromyalgia, neuropathic pain, or other chronic pain

Common class adverse effects

- Similar to those above for SSRIs; but also, with added risk of **increasing blood pressure/HTN**, hyponatremia, and dizziness
- **Black box warning**: increased **suicidality** in **children/adolescents/young adults** (<25 y.o.)

Norepinephrine Reuptake Inhibitors (NRI)

- Used to treat MDD, anxiety, panic disorder, ADHD, narcolepsy, obesity (appetite suppressant)
  - MOA: Block the action of the NE transporter
- Atomoxetine (Strattera)
  - Blocks NE reuptake pumps, increases DA in prefrontal cortex
  - Successful non-stimulant treatment of **ADHD** (more info in non-stimulant section)
  - Used as alterative to stimulants for ADHD (common choice for those with cooccurring anxiety or substance abuse history)
  - Dosed by weight
  - Rare side effect: priapism

- Contraindicated in patients with pheochromocytoma
  - May notice symptom improvement in ADHD as early as first day
  - Takes 2-4 weeks for full efficacy
  - FDA approved for ADHD in adults and children; used off-label for treatment-resistant depression

- Viloxazine (Vivalan/Qelbree)
  - May cause increased ESR, EKG changes, tremor
  - Block NE reuptake pumps, 5HT reuptake; has antagonist action at 5HT2B, agonist action at 5HT2C that increases 5HT levels; increases both DA and NE in prefrontal cortex
  - Dosing adjustment indicated in renal insufficiency
  - Not recommended for use in patients with hepatic insufficiency
  - FDA approved for ADHD ages 6 and up; used off-label for MDD

- Maprotiline (Ludiomil)
  - Block NE reuptake pump, more potent at NE than 5HT reuptake pumps
  - Also classified as a TCA
  - Dose-related increased risk of seizures
  - QTc prolongation risk
  - Contraindicated in patients with history of QTc prolongation or arrhythmia, recent myocardial infarction heart failure
  - FDA approved depression; used off-label for anxiety, neuropathic and chronic pain, treatment-resistant depression

Common class adverse effects

- Generally well tolerated, but headache, dry mouth, **loss of appetite**, fatigue, nausea, and vomiting may occur
- Serious side effects include suicidality (black box warning) and withdrawal

Norepinephrine and Dopamine Reuptake Inhibitors (NDRI)

- Used to treat MDD, SAD, nicotine addiction, bipolar disorder, ADHD
  - MOA: Block NE and dopamine from being transported back into the cells that released them, causing a greater number of NE and dopamine to be available

- Bupropion (Wellbutrin)
  - Only FDA approved NDRI to treat depression
  - Effective for **smoking cessation**
  - **Lowers seizure threshold** (CI in patients with seizure disorder);
    - **Avoid in those with eating disorders/bulimia** (vomiting can also lower seizure threshold due to electrolyte imbalances);

- Used off label for anxiety but is initially activating, which can sometimes worsen symptoms of anxiety
- Commonly used for treatment of ADHD
- May be added to SSRIs for SSRI-induced sexual dysfunction or SSRI-induced apathy
- FDA approved for MDD, Seasonal Affective disorder (SAD), nicotine addiction; used off-label for ADHD in adults, bipolar depression, sexual dysfunction

- Common adverse effects
  - Insomnia, weight loss, anxiety, dizziness, sweating, **HTN**, **seizures, cardiotoxicity**

<u>Tricyclic Antidepressants (TCAs)</u>

- Used for insomnia, MDD, neuropathic pain, migraine
  - MOA: Inhibit neuronal reuptake of serotonin and 5HT, NE, alpha 1, anticholinergic, histamine, Na+
    - Block H1 histamine receptor, anticholinergic, alpha-1 antagonist, and Na+ channels
  - Takes **4-6 weeks** to reach therapeutic effects
  - Highly lethal in overdose given QTc prolongation, cardiac dysrhythmias, severe hypotension, convulsions; use in caution with patients with history of suicidality
  - Combination of TCAs + anticholinergic medications can result in paralytic ileus, hyperthermia
  - Monitor weight during use
  - Avoid alcohol use

- Amitriptyline (Elavil)
  - Commonly used for migraine prophylaxis
  - Used for pain including, including IBS related pain, as well insomnia
  - FDA approved for depression; used off-label for chronic headache prevention, neuropathic or chronic pain, fibromyalgia, insomnia, treatment-resistant depression

- Doxepin (Silenor)
  - At antidepressant doses (75-150 mg/day) mechanism of action is blockade of 5HT, NE reuptake
  - At hypnotic doses (3-6 mg/day) has potent blockage of H1 receptors, decreasing wakefulness and promoting sleep
    - Commonly used at a low dose for insomnia
  - FDA approved for insomnia, depression, psychotic depression with anxiety; used off-label for anxiety, neuropathic or chronic pain, treatment-resistant depression

- Imipramine (Tofranil)
  - Preferred TCA for enuresis

  - FDA approved for depression; used off-label for anxiety, treatment-resistant depression, neuropathic or chronic pain, insomnia, enuresis

- Nortriptyline (Pamelor)
  - FDA approved for MDD; used off-label for anxiety, insomnia, treatment-resistant depression, neuropathic or chronic pain

- Desipramine (Norpramin)
  - May have less anticholinergic activity than other TCAs; may have less sedative, dry mouth, constipation, blurred vision side effects
  - FDA approved for depression; used off-label for anxiety, neuropathic or chronic pain, insomnia, treatment-resistant depression
- Amoxapine (Ascendin)
  - May have faster onset of action than other antidepressants
  - May cause akathisia, drug-induced parkinsonism at high doses, and long-term high-dose use is associated with risk of tardive dyskinesia
  - FDA approved for depression; used off-label for anxiety, insomnia, treatment-resistant depression, neuropathic or chronic pain

Common class adverse effects

  - Less commonly used due to toxicity triad (**cardiotoxicity, convulsions, coma**), overdose, anticholinergic symptoms, postural hypotension, **QTc prolongation** that may lead to torsades de pointe, weight gain
  - For TCA overdose with QRS prolongation - **treat with sodium bicarbonate** to increase extracellular sodium concentration

Monoamine Oxidase Inhibitors (MAOIs)

- **Not** commonly used, not first line due to **many drug and food interactions**; used for refractory depression/anxiety
  - MOA: Blocks the breakdown of dopamine, serotonin, epinephrine, and NE by inhibiting monoamine oxidase
  - Begins to have an effect in 10-14 days

- Phenelzine (Nardil) Non-selective
  - FDA approved for treatment-resistant depression, panic disorder, social anxiety disorder

- Selegiline (Emsam)
  - **MAO-B selectivity** so less chance of HTN crisis; Comes in **patch form**
  - FDA approved for Parkinson disease; transdermal patch is approved for MDD

- Tranylcypromine (Parnate) Non-selective

- May have some stimulant effects, as structurally similar to amphetamine
- FDA approved for MDD; used off-label for treatment-resistant depression

Common class adverse effects

- **Hypertensive crisis with sympathomimetics or foods high in tyramine** (aged cheese, wine, beer, smoked meat, coffee, tea, chocolate), insomnia, anxiety, weight gain, orthostasis
- Contraindicated to give MAOI and SSRI → serotonin syndrome
- Contraindicated to give MAOI and TCA → Causes delirium and hypertension

Atypical Anti-Depressants

- Nefazodone (Serzone)
    - Removed from most non-US markets due to liver injury

- Trazodone (Desyrel/Molipaxin)
    - MOA: Serotonin modulator that antagonizes postsynaptic 5HT-2 receptors and inhibits serotonin uptake. Also causes alpha-1 to blockade
    - Indicated for depression, but commonly used for **insomnia**
    - Serotonin receptor antagonists and reuptake inhibitors (SARI)
    - Adverse effects include vasodilation (priapism MC second to alpha blockade), sedation, serotonin syndrome, sexual dysfunction
    - **Avoid in sickle cell patients and those with multiple myeloma** as it may cause occlusive crisis in those select patient populations. CI with benzos and barbiturates
    - FDA approved for depression; used off-label for insomnia, anxiety
    - Contraindicated to use with benzodiazepines, barbiturates given risk for respiratory depression

- Mirtazapine (Remeron)
    - MOA: Alpha-2 antagonist which causes increased serotonin and NE in the synapse. Also blocks 5HT2 and 5HT3 receptors
    - MC used for MDD and insomnia
    - Adverse effects include weight gain (potent H1 blocker), **sedation**, constipation, agranulocytosis, dry mouth. Little to no sexual dysfunction
        - Good for anorexia due to weight gain SE
    - Use with caution with MAOIs
    - FDA approved for MDD; used off-label for GAD, panic disorder, PTSD

- Vortioxetine (Brintellix/Trintellix)

- SSRI/5-HT_{1A} Receptor Partial Agonist/5-HT_3 Antagonist
  - Directly affects multiple serotonin receptors in addition to inhibiting the reuptake of serotonin
  - Indicated for depression, but used off-label for anxiety as well
  - Thought to have less weight gain and sexual side effects than traditional SSRIs
  - FDA approved for MDD; used off-label for GAD, may have some benefit for cognitive symptoms associated with depression, geriatric depression

- Vilazodone (Viibryd)
  - SSRI/5-HT_{1A} Receptor Partial Agonist
    - Indicated for depression and used off label for anxiety
    - ADRs similar to Vortioxetine
  - May begin to show benefit in the first week
  - FDA approved for MDD; used off-label for anxiety, OCD

Postpartum Depression (PPD)

- SSRIs are generally used for initial treatment of moderate to severe PPD
- SNRIs and TCAs have also been used with limited evidence
- Brexanolone (Zulresso),
  - MOA: $GABA_A$ receptor modulator
  - First drug to be approved by the FDA specifically for treatment of PPD
  - 60-hour IV infusion
- Zuranolone (Zurzuvae)
  - MOA: $GABA_A$ receptor modulator
  - First once daily oral formulation for PPD

Alternative Therapies

Refractory Depression Treatment

- **Electro-Convulsive Therapy (ECT)**
  - Indications: **Atypical depression, depression refractory to medication and/or psychotherapy, depression with psychosis, acutely suicidal patients**
    - Safe in elderly and pregnant populations
    - has the highest rates of response and remission of any form of antidepressant therapy (70-90%)
    - Procedure: Patient is sedated with general anesthesia and muscle relaxants to limit movement. Electrodes are placed on the scalp and an electric current is passed through the

electrode. It is NOT painful as the current is not detectable. The procedure lasts a total of 5-10 minutes
    - Typical course of treatment: 3 times per week for a total of 6-12 treatments
    - Adverse effects include **headaches**, muscle aches, GI upset, **memory loss** that improves over time (more common with traditional ECT where electrodes are placed on both sides of the head vs unilateral ECT which is less likely to cause memory loss)

- **Repetitive Transcranial Magnetic Stimulation (rTMS)**
  - Indications: Atypical depression, depression refractory to medication and/or psychotherapy, depression with psychosis, acutely suicidal patients
    - Safe in elderly and pregnant populations
    - Procedure: An electromagnetic coil is placed on the scalp near the forehead and the magnet delivers a magnetic pulse to stimulate nerves in the mood centers of the brain
    - Typical course of treatment: 4-5 times a week for 4-6 weeks
    - Adverse effects include headache, scalp discomfort at site of stimulation, spasms of facial muscles, lightheadedness, hearing loss (patients require ear protection during procedure)

- **Vagus Nerve Stimulation (VNS)**
  - Indications: Epilepsy and intense depression that is refractory to treatment
  - Procedure: A device is implanted under the skin on the chest with a wire connecting the device to the **left vagus nerve**. Upon activation, a signal is sent from the vagus nerve to the brain. (Note: right vagus nerve carries fibers to the heart)
  - Adverse effects include that of surgery (pain, infection) as well as vocal cord paralysis, voice hoarseness, cough, throat pain, shortness of breath, difficulty swallowing

- **Deep Brain Stimulation (DBS)**
  - Indications: Dystonia, epilepsy, OCD, Parkinson's disease, addiction, essential tremor, dementia, depression, Huntington's disease, multiple sclerosis
  - Procedure: Implantation of electrodes within certain areas of the brain which produce electrical impulses to help regulate abnormal pulses
  - Adverse effects: Risks of surgery (pain, infection) as well as bleeding, stroke, heart problems, seizures, etc.

- **Ketamine/Esketamine**

- Anti-depressant; General Anesthetic; also used for PTSD
- MOA: NMDA receptor antagonist that blocks glutamate. Direct action on the cortex and limbic system → a cataleptic-like state in which the patient is dissociated from their surroundings.
- Available in IV, intranasal and sublingual formulations
- Frequency of treatment varies by formulation and individual protocols

- **Bright Light Therapy**
  - Not FDA approved; used off-label for Seasonal Affective disorder (SAD)
  - May work by stimulating the retina, optic nerve which has projection to hypothalamic suprachiasmatic nucleus, inhibiting melatonin production
  - Thought to be most effective for patients presenting with atypical depression symptoms
  - Minimum intensity of light required is 10,000 lux, administered about 24 inches from patient for about 30 minutes after waking
  - Side effects: headaches

Benzodiazepines

- Schedule IV **controlled substances**. Consider getting a UDS prior to rx of any controlled substance; Risk of addiction/tolerance/abuse
- MOA: **Binds to GABA receptors** which increases frequency of chloride channel opening, causing hyperpolarization of the neurons and depression of the central nervous system
  - Similar to the MOA of alcohol
- Metabolism
  - Hepatic (use with caution in those with cirrhosis or liver failure)
- Indications for prescribing benzodiazepines
  - **1st line for status epilepticus** (defer to neurology)
  - **1st line for alcohol withdrawal**
  - Used for conscious sedation for minor procedures such as TEE, colonoscopy, etc. as benzos cause muscle relaxation and sedation
  - **Anxiety**
    - **Not** 1st line but can be used for episodic anxiety/panic attacks
    - Daily use not recommended
    - Better for episodic anxiety (ex. fear of airplanes) as opposed to generalized anxiety (SSRI first line)
  - **Panic disorder**
    - Can be used for acute episodic panic attacks, but SSRIs better for prevention (so patient does not reach panic threshold to begin

with, as opposed to just aborting the panic attack after it has occurred)

Commonly used BDZ	Onset	Half-life (hrs)	Considerations
Alprazolam (Xanax)	Fast	6- 15 hr	Used for panic attacks
Chlordiazepoxide (Librium)	Intermediate	8-28 hr	Used for alcohol withdrawal
Clonazepam (Klonopin)	Slow	18-50 hr	Frequently abused
Diazepam (Valium)	Fast	20-50 hr	Used to aid in tapering off of other benzo's due to the long half-life. Fat soluble (less predictable).
Lorazepam (Ativan)	Fast	5-8 hr	Used for panic attacks
Midazolam (Versed)	Very fast	1-4 hr	Used for sedation (adults/kids)

Common class adverse effects

- **Tolerance/addiction/abuse**
- CNS depression
- Anterograde amnesia
- Paradoxical agitation
- Poor sleep (less REM); associated with **earlier onset of dementia**
- Risk of withdrawal
  - **Avoid daily/long-term use**. If on long-term, d/c requires a **taper** to avoid withdrawal/adverse effects (withdrawal can result in **death**)

- **Do not use in conjunction with alcohol, anticholinergics, barbiturates, sedatives, neuroleptics**
- **Fatal** in overdose; fatal at a lower dose when combined with alcohol/other substances
  - Hence small quantities prescribed at a time
- For overdose → **Flumazenil** is the drug of choice as it is a competitive antagonist for GABA

Editor's note – There is a high risk of dependence and abuse with benzodiazepines, and in the aftermath of the opioid epidemic there is a renewed attention paid to the prescribing of such medications. It is our responsibility to act as judicious stewards, doing our best to avoid prescribing these medications when unnecessary while also prescribing them, when necessary, with careful attention to educating the patient on all side effects, risks, and alternative options.

Sleep-Related Medications

Sedative Hypnotics (non-benzodiazepine sedatives)

- Schedule IV **controlled substances**. Consider getting a UDS prior to rx of any controlled substance; Risk of addiction/tolerance/abuse
- MOA: Bind to GABA at the same site as benzodiazepines
  - Commonly used for **insomnia**
  - Metabolism hepatic (use with caution in cirrhosis or liver failure)

- Zolpidem (Ambien)
  - Indicated for the short-term treatment of insomnia characterized by difficulties falling asleep
  - Increased falls and ataxia in the elderly
  - Gender based dosing. Initial dosing of ER formulation 6.25 mg (females) or 6.25 to 12.5 mg (males), and initial dosing of IR formulation is 5 mg (females) or 5 to 10 mg (males)
  - Infamous for sleep walking/sleep driving

- Zaleplon (Sonata)
  - Similar to Zolpidem, with slightly fewer drug to drug interactions
- Eszopiclone (Lunesta)
  - Longer acting than. Zolpidem and Zaleplon
- **Common class adverse effects**
  - **Tolerance/addiction/abuse**
  - CNS depression
  - Poor sleep (less REM); associated with **earlier onset of dementia**
  - + the same as benzodiazepines but there is less of an anxiolytic and anticonvulsant effect and therefore these are used to help patients sleep.
    - Lower risk of tolerance/withdrawal as compared to benzodiazepines

- For overdose → **Flumazenil** is the drug of choice as it is a competitive antagonist for GABA

Dual-Orexin Receptor Antagonists (DORAs)

- Schedule IV **controlled substances**. Consider getting a UDS prior to rx of any controlled substance; Risk of addiction/tolerance/abuse
- MOA: Orexin antagonist
  - Commonly used for **insomnia**

- Suvorexant (Belsomra)

- Indicated for the treatment of insomnia, characterized by difficulties falling or staying asleep

- Daridorexant (Quviviq)

- Lemborexant (Dayvigo)

Non-benzodiazepines Sedatives → Melatonin Receptor Agonists

- MOA: Binds to melatonin receptors (MT-1 and MT-2) in the suprachiasmatic nucleus
    - No effect on GABA

- Ramelteon (Rozerem)
    - Indicated for treatment of **insomnia**
    - **Not** a controlled substance – said to have limited risk for abuse and not habit-forming
    - Adverse effects – dizziness and drowsiness

Other medications commonly given for sleep

- Melatonin
    - OTC supplement; good to start here but not effective for everyone

- Hydroxyzine
    - antihistamine

- Prazosin
    - antihypertensive, monitor BP; used for PTSD-associated nightmares

Editor's notes –
1) Make sure patient first trials sleep hygiene (cool/quiet/dark sleep conditions, avoid blue light and caffeine closer to bedtime, etc.) and CBT which can also be helpful for sleep
2) Rule out other conditions/structural causes of sleep disturbance, i.e. sleep apnea
3) If other conditions such as anxiety for example are disturbing sleep, treating anxiety with SSRI can also resolve sleep issues oftentimes
4) If patients have co-occurring mood disorder(s) along with insomnia, you can specifically choose an existing pharmacological treatment option for their mood disorder that is also sedating (ex. quetiapine or olanzapine for those with bipolar disorder). Then they can take it before bed and the medication helps stabilize their mood and the sedating side effect can help their insomnia/sleep disturbance all with one agent.

Barbiturates

- **Controlled substances.** Consider getting a UDS prior to rx of any controlled substance; Risk of addiction/tolerance/abuse
  - *Note – this class in not commonly used clinically in psychiatry*
- MOA: Binds to GABA at an allosteric site that is different than that of benzodiazepines. These keep the chloride channels open longer (longer half-life) and therefore are <u>more addictive</u>
- Potent CYP-450 metabolism
  - Use with caution in combo with many other drugs

- Thiopental sodium (Pentothal)
  - Commonly used for rapid sequence intubation (lasts 30 seconds to 5 minutes

- Phenobarbital
  - Used for status epilepticus as last line treatment
  - Causes hypotension and hypo-respiration

- Primidone (Myosoline)
  - Used for essential tremor
  - Adverse effects include severe hypotension and hypo-respiration; therefore these are commonly used when intubating patients/surgery induction and seizure disorders/status epilepticus
  - Avoid in the elderly

Antipsychotics

Treat psychosis, all forms of schizophrenia, psychotic ideations, drug-induced psychosis, psychotic depression, acute mania, bipolar disorder, treatment resistant depression, and other behavioral issues

Typical antipsychotics (1st Generation)

- Used especially for positive symptoms of schizophrenia (hallucinations and delusions)
- MOA: Block central dopamine receptors

- Chlorprom**azine** (Thorazine)
  - Known for sedation and orthostatic hypotension
  - Reduces efficacy of anticoagulants
  - FDA approved for schizophrenia, acute psychosis; often used off-label for bipolar disorder

- Thiorid**azine** (Mellaril)

- Increased incidence of QT prolongation & retinitis pigmentosa
- CYP2D6 inhibitors can raise levels of thioridazine (ex: paroxetine, fluoxetine, duloxetine, bupropion, sertraline, citalopram, etc.)
- FDA approved for second-line treatment of schizophrenia

- Fluphen**azine** (Prolixin)
  - Available in long-acting intramuscular form
  - Use with caution in renal, hepatic, cardiac impairment populations
  - FDA approved for psychotic disorders; used off-label for bipolar disorder

- Trifluoper**azine** (Stelazine)
  - Contraindicated in bone marrow depression, liver disease
  - If used with propranolol, can increase levels of both medications
  - FDA approved for schizophrenia, non-psychotic anxiety; used off-label for other psychotic disorders, bipolar disorder

- Perphen**azine** (Trilafon)
  - FDA approved for schizophrenia and for the control of severe nausea and vomiting in adults

- Thiothixene (Navane)
  - FDA approved for schizophrenia; used off-label for other psychotic disorders, bipolar disorder

- Loxapine (Loxitane)
  - Less weight gain associated than other antipsychotics
  - FDA approved for schizophrenia, acute treatment of agitation of schizophrenia or bipolar disorder
- Pimozide (Orap)
  - Dose-dependent QTc prolongation; start low and go slow
  - Xontraindicated with use of macrolide antibiotics, azole antifungal agents given inhibition of pimozide metabolism
  - CYP450 3A4 inhibitors (fluoxetine, sertraline, fluvoxamine, nefazodone, grapefruit juice) can increase levels
  - FDA approved for suppression of motor, phonic tics in patients with Tourette syndrome as second-line treatment; used off-label for psychotic disorders as second-line treatment

- Haloperidol (Haldol)
  - FDA approved for psychotic disorders, Tourette's syndrome motor, phonic tics; often used off-label for bipolar disorder, behavioral disturbances in dementia, delirium
  - EPS syndromes are very common
  - Contraindicated in Parkinson's disease

- CYP450 2D6 and 3A4 metabolism, so many medication interactions

Common class adverse effects

- Sedation
- Extrapyramidal symptoms **(EPS)**
    - Tardive Dyskinesia (TD)- **Late onset development of involuntary, choreoathetoid movements** of tongue, lower face, jaw, and extremities that **develops years after starting** an antipsychotic agent, especially 1st generation medications
    - Responds to VMAT inhibitors (**deuterobenzene and valbenazine**)
    - May be irreversible
    - Abnormal Involuntary Movement Scale (AIMS) assessment can be used to help assess

- Neuroleptic Malignant Syndrome (NMS)- Medical emergency consisting of autonomic instability (vital signs unstable), muscle rigidity, tremors, fever, diaphoresis, delirium that can occur at any time after starting antipsychotics, especially 1st generation
    - Mechanism: Increased white blood cells, increase CPK, and increase liver enzymes lead to muscle breakdown, causing autonomic instability
    - Responds to **bromocriptine** (dopamine agonist) and **dantrolene sodium** (muscle relaxer that inhibits calcium release into the sarcoplasmic reticulum)
- Anticholinergic effects
    - Dry mouth, constipation, urinary retention, bowel obstruction, dilated pupils, blurred vision, increased heart rate, and decreased sweating

- Endocrine effects
    - Increased prolactin levels
        - Galactorrhea
        - Gynecomastia
        - Sexual dysfunction
        - Weight gain

- Cardiovascular effects
    - Hypotension
    - QTc interval prolongation

Atypical antipsychotics (2nd Generation [SgA's])

- Widely used and effective to treat **psychosis**, both positive and negative symptoms of schizophrenia, bipolar disorder/**mania**

- *Clinically second-generation antipsychotics are more commonly used than first generation antipsychotics*

- All also indicated as adjunct **MDD treatment**
  - Negative symptoms include lack of motivation, slow movement, poor grooming, reduced range of emotion, among others.
  - 1st line for the treatment of schizophrenia due to the better side effect profile
  - Also effective in treating bipolar type 1 and treatment resistant depression
  - **MOA:** Block central dopamine and serotonin receptors

"The Pines" 5HT2A action > D2

- Olanza<u>pine</u> (Zyprexa)
  - Helps with sleep, but known to cause **weight gain**
  - Higher risk for type 2 diabetes, dyslipidemia
  - Dose may need adjusted down with CYP1A2 inducers (ex: cigarette smoke)
  - FDA approved for acute agitation in schizophrenia, acute mania/mixed mania as monotherapy or adjunctive treatment in bipolar disorder, bipolar maintenance, bipolar depression, treatment-resistant depression as adjunctive agent; used off-label in other psychotic disorders, behavioral disturbances, PTSD, Borderline Personality disorder

- Olanza<u>pine</u> + samidorphan (Lybalvi)
  - The added samidorphan helps *negate the weight gain of olanzapine*

- Quetia<u>pine</u> (Seroquel)
  - Frequently used off-label as a sleep aid and for anxiety, often at low doses
  - Dizziness and sedation common
  - Higher doses (>400 mg) most effective for mania, psychosis symptoms
  - Minimal motor side effects, prolactin elevation
  - FDA approved for acute and maintenance treatments of schizophrenia, acute mania, bipolar depression, bipolar maintenance, Major depressive disorder; used off-label for other psychotic disorders, mixed mania episodes, severe treatment-resistant anxiety, PTSD, behavioral disturbances/psychosis associated w/ Parkinson's Lewy body dementia
- Asena<u>pine</u> (Saphris)
  - Contraindicated in severe hepatic impairment
  - Inhibits CYP2D6, can increase levels of beta blockers
  - CYP1A2 inhibitors can increase levels of Asenapine (ex: fluvoxamine)

    - FDA approved for schizophrenia, acute mania/mixed mania as monotherapy or adjunctive agent, bipolar maintenance; used off-label for behavioral disturbances in dementia, other psychotic disorders, bipolar depression, treatment-resistant depression

- Clozapine (Clozaril)
    - Primarily used inpatient
    - Known for metabolic syndrome and **agranulocytosis –monitor CBCs**
    - Considered gold-standard treatment for treatment-resistant schizophrenia
    - Trough plasma levels used for monitoring; threshold for response is generally 350 ng/mL
    - Distribution managed by Risk Evaluation and Mitigation Strategy (REMS) program
    - CYP1A2 /2D6 inhibitors can markedly increase the level of clozapine and dose must be decreased
    - CYP450 1A2 inducers, such as cigarette smoke, can decrease plasma levels of clozapine – close monitoring needed, dose reductions indicated for patients who are quitting smoking
    - CYP3A4 inhibitors (ex: ketoconazole) can increase plasma levels significantly
    - Can improve negative as well as positive symptoms of schizophrenia
    - FDA approved for treatment resistant schizophrenia, reducing suicidality in patients with schizophrenia and schizoaffective disorder; used off-label for treatment-resistant bipolar disorder, aggression

"The Dones"

- Risperidone (Risperdal)
    - Dose-dependent risk for drug-induced parkinsonism, akathisia, hyperprolactinemia
    - Highest risk of hyperprolactinemia among antipsychotic medications
    - FDA approved for schizophrenia, other psychotic disorders, acute/mixed mania, bipolar maintenance as monotherapy or adjunctive, Autism-related irritability in children aged 5-16; used off-label for bipolar depression, treatment-resistant depression, PTSD, behavioral disturbances in dementia

- Ziprasidone (Geodon)
    - Must be taken with food for medication to be bioavailable
    - May be activating at low doses
    - Greater risk for QTc prolongation than other antipsychotics
    - Less weight gain associated than most other atypical antipsychotics
    - FDA approved for schizophrenia, acute mania/mixed mania, and bipolar maintenance; used off-label for other psychotic disorders,

refractory depression, and PTSD

- Lurasidone (Latuda)
  - Must be taken with food for medication to be bioavailable
  - Contraindicated with strong CYP3A4 inhibitors (ex: ketoconazole) or inducers (ex: phenytoin)
  - FDA approved for schizophrenia, bipolar depression; used off-label for other psychotic disorders, treatment-resistant depression, PTSD

- Paliperidone (Invega)
  - Dose-dependent risk for drug-induced parkinsonism
  - Higher risk for hyperprolactinemia than other atypical antipsychotics
  - QTc prolongation risk higher than other antipsychotics
  - Long-acting formulations including every 6-month option
  - FDA approved for schizophrenia, schizoaffective disorder; used off-label for other psychotic disorder, acute mania/mixed mania and bipolar maintenance, treatment-resistant depression

- Iloperidone (Fanapt)
  - Dose-dependent risk for tachycardia
  - QTc prolongation risk higher than other antipsychotic agents
  - FDA approved for schizophrenia; used off-label for other psychotic disorders, bipolar depression, bipolar maintenance, treatment-resistant depression

"Two PIPS and a RIP" D2 > 5HT2A action

- Aripiprazole (Abilify)
  - Commonly used medication
  - FDA approved for schizophrenia (ages 13+), bipolar maintenance, acute mania/mixed mania, Major depressive disorder (adjunctive agent), Autism-rclated irritability in children, Tourette's disorder; used off-label for other psychotic disorders, bipolar depression, OCD (as adjunct agent to SSRIs)

- Brexpiprazole (Rexulti)
  - Partial agonist at D2, 5HT1A, antagonism of 5HT2A
  - Dose-dependent risk for akathisia, restlessness
  - FDA approved for schizophrenia, Major depressive disorder (adjunct), agitation associated with Alzheimer's disease; used off-label for other psychotic disorders, bipolar depression, acute/mixed mania, bipolar maintenance

- Cariprazine (Vraylar)
  - Helpful for positive and negative symptoms of psychosis, mood instability

- Partial agonism at D2, 5HT1A, antagonism at 5HT2A and 5HT2B
- FDA approved for schizophrenia, acute/mixed mania, bipolar depression, Major depressive disorder (adjunct); used off-label for other psychotic disorders, bipolar maintenance, negative symptoms of schizophrenia

Common class adverse effects

- EPS, TD, and NMS; however considerably lower incidence than typical antipsychotics
- Sexual dysfunction
- Can elevate TSH
- Hyperprolactinemia
- Metabolic syndrome including higher risk for diabetes, weight gain, hyperlipidemia
  - Metformin sometimes given in conjunction with second-generation antipsychotics to combat weight gain
- Routine lab monitoring – CBC, CMP/lipid panel, HbA1c, TSH, prolactin

Extrapyramidal side effects of antipsychotics

- Acute Dystonia – **Painful, abnormal, prolonged contractions of the muscles** that develop within hours to days of starting or increasing doses of antipsychotics. Occurs in eyes (oculogyric crisis), head/neck (torticollis), limbs and trunk. More common with 1st generation class
  - Add **Cogentin or Benadryl** to reduce, prevent, or avoid dystonia from occurring
  - Risk factors include young age, male gender, and high doses of meds

- Parkinsonism – Triad of resting tremors ("pill-rolling"), muscular rigidity (cogwheel), and bradykinesia/akinesia. May also be associated with shuffling gait, drooling, and rabbit syndrome (tremor of perioral muscles). Develops within days to weeks of staring or increasing dose of antipsychotics, particularly the 1st generation
  - Responds to amantadine and anticholinergics
  - Risk factors include older age and female gender

- Akathisia **(MC EPS symptom)** – Subjective feeling of restlessness, anxiety, pacing, or frequent sitting/standing/movement
  - Responds to beta blockers and benzodiazepines
  - Older females may be at an increased risk

- Tardive Dyskinesia – **Late onset development of involuntary, choreoathetoid movements** of tongue, lower face, jaw, and extremities that **develops years after starting** an antipsychotic agent, especially 1st generation medications

- Responds to VMAT inhibitors (**deuterobenzene and valbenazine**)
- May be irreversible

- Neuroleptic Malignant Syndrome (NMS) – **Medical emergency** consisting of autonomic instability (**vital signs unstable**), muscle rigidity, tremors, fever, diaphoresis, delirium that can occur at any time after starting antipsychotics, especially 1st generation
  - Mechanism: Increased white blood cells, increase CPK, and increase liver enzymes lead to muscle breakdown, causing autonomic instability
  - Responds to **bromocriptine** (dopamine agonist) and **dantrolene sodium** (muscle relaxer that inhibits calcium release into the sarcoplasmic reticulum)

Mood Stabilizers

- Lithium
  - **Used for Bipolar I Disorder** (also used for adjunct therapy for depression)
  - **MOA:** Stimulates the NMDA receptor and increases glutamate at the postsynaptic neuron
  - Adverse effects include nausea, tremor, **polyuria/diabetes insipidus, hypothyroidism, cardiac dysrhythmias**, weight gain, thirst, acne, edema, leukocytosis, **teratogenic** potential
  - Routine lab monitoring – CBC, CMP, TSH, BUN/Cr (**renally cleared medication**), hCG (teratogenic), lithium, level; ECG
  - **Lithium has a narrow therapeutic index** → check lithium levels to confirm safe/effective dosing
  - Reduces suicidality, suicide risk
  - Renally cleared; be aware of medications that may decrease renal clearance (ex: metronidazole
  - Toxicity symptoms of tremor, diarrhea, vomiting, sedation, ataxia
    - Treated with dialysis, aggressive oral and IV hydration
  - Side effects may include memory impairment, weight gain, hair loss
  - Absorption decreased on an empty stomach
  - Contraindicated with severe renal disease, cardiovascular disease, Brugada syndrome
  - Many drug interactions, including NSAIDs, selective COX-2 inhibitors, ACEIs, CCBs, can increase plasma levels and toxicity risk
  - Teratogen: cardiac malformations
  - FDA approved for mania, maintenance of bipolar disorder; used off-label for bipolar depression, Major depressive disorder

Anticonvulsants (as mood stabilizers)

- Valproic acid (Depakote)
  - Good for rapidly cycling disorders between mania and depression
  - MOA: Opens chloride channels, **blocks sodium channels, and increases GABA**
  - Adverse effects include **thrombocytopenia**, pancreatitis, hair loss, weight gain, GI dysfunction, **teratogenic – neural tube defects (avoid in women of childbearing age)**
  - Routine labs CBC w/ diff, LFT + amylase, **hCG (teratogenic)**
  - FDA approved for acute/mixed mania, maintenance treatment of bipolar disorder; used off-label for bipolar depression, psychosis, schizophrenia

- Carbamazepine
  - MOA: Inhibit firing via inactivating Na+ channels; **Potent CYP450 inducer**
  - Adverse effects include nausea, vomiting, agranulocytosis, increased LFTs, slurred speech, drowsiness, **teratogenic** potential
  - Routine labs CBC w/ diff, iron levels, LFTs + amylase, hCG
  - Teratogenic
  - FDA approved for acute/mixed mania episodes; used off-label for bipolar depression, bipolar maintenance, psychosis, schizophrenia

- Lamotrigine (Lamictal) - common mood stabilizer **maintenance therapy for bipolar disorder**
  - MOA: Selectively binds sodium channels and inhibits release of glutamate
  - Adverse effects include leukopenia**, rash - Stevens Johnson Syndrome risk,** hepatitis, N/V/D, sleep, dizziness
  - Titrate up slowly/taper off slowly to minimize SJS risk
  - FDA approved for maintenance of Bipolar I; used off-label for bipolar depression, mania, psychosis, schizophrenia, neuropathic pain, chronic pain
  - Teratogenic

- Gabapentin (Neurontin)
  - Controlled substance in select states only – some potential for abuse
  - MOA: Has a high affinity for voltage gated calcium channels and in turn, inhibits the release of excitatory neurotransmitters
  - Adverse effects include somnolence, ataxia, fatigue, weight gain
  - Used frequently in patients with coexisting anxiety

- Topiramate (Topamax)

- MOA: Blocks sodium and calcium channels while also inhibiting the effect of GABA
- Adverse effects include memory problems, fatigue

ADHD Treatments

Stimulant Medications

- Schedule II **controlled substances** (high potential for abuse/addiction; recognized medical use). Consider getting a UDS prior to rx of any controlled substance.
- Used as first-line treatment for ADHD.
  - Two stimulant classes, methylphenidates and amphetamines, both medications are available in a variety of formulations and offer similar efficacy
  - MOA: Achieve effects via increasing **NE and dopamine activity**
  - Metabolism → **Metabolized by the liver and excreted via the kidneys,** potential for nephrotoxicity especially in overdose

Methylphenidate Class

- Methylphenidate (immediate and extended-release formulations)
  - Methylphenidate Long Acting (Ritalin/Metadate)
    - Ritalin LA is 50% immediate release and 50% extended release, whereas Metadate CD is 30% immediate release and 70% extended release. Metadate is ideal for patients whose symptoms are worse later in the day than they are at the start of it.
    - Both are said to last up to 8 hours (metabolism varies by patient)
    - Capsules that can be opened and sprinkled into food
      - Note – should not be used in lactose intolerant patients
  - Methylphenidate HCl (Concerta)
    - Longer acting, up to 12 hours
  - Methylphenidate HCl (Journay PM)
    - Taken at night, and begins to work 8 hours later.
    - Ideal for children with symptoms from the moment they awake
  - Methylphenidate patch (Daytrana) Long-acting
    - Helpful in younger children who will not take medication
  - Methylphenidate Long Acting Chewable (Quillichew ER)
  - Methylphenidate Long-Acting Liquid (Quillivant XR)

- Dexmethylphenidate (Focalin), available in short and long acting

- Stronger than methylphenidate

Amphetamine Class

- Amphetamine
  - Comes in long-acting Liquid (Dyanavel/Adzenys), Chewable (Dyanavel), ODT (Adzenys), Super-long-acting capsule (Mydayis)

- Amphetamine-Dextroamphetamine (immediate and extended-release formulations)
  - Mixed amphetamine salts (Adderall)
- Dextroamphetamine
  - Long-acting oral formulation (Dexedrine Spansule), long-acting patch (Xelstrym), Chewable (Dyanavel long-acting and Zenzedi short-acting), short-acting liquid (ProCentra)

- Lisdexamfetamine dimesylate (Vyvanse)
  - Amphetamine w/ lysine → requires GI metabolization and therefore thought to be **lower risk for abuse than other stimulant choices** (if snorted medication would cause no effect)
  - Due to this GI absorption, it takes longer to work, and lasts for up to 14 hours.
  - Only approved in individuals ≥6 years old
  - Additional indication for binge eating disorder w/ or w/o ADHD diagnosis
    - *Sometimes seen as having superior side effect profile to other stimulants, commonly with a smoother release/" come down"*

- **General stimulant adverse effects**
  - The labels of all stimulants contain a boxed warning about the high risk of **abuse and dependence** associated with these drugs; patients should be monitored for signs of abuse. Do not use in those with history of drug abuse.
    - Routine UDSs commonly done
  - *In general, stimulants have risk for the similar side effects. At times different formulations/changing classes may be tolerated better clinically, but this varies for each individual patient.*
  - **Raise BP & HR**
    - Avoid in those with cardiovascular issues or arrythmias
    - **ECG** helpful prior to initiation
  - **Sleep disruption**
  - **Loss of appetite**
    - Common side effect. Monitor growth and ensure caloric intake goals are met.

    - When weight goals are not maintained but dose cannot be lowered Cyproheptadine (first gen antihistamine) can be added for appetite stimulation
  - Nervousness/anxiety
    - In some patients, stimulants can increase/worsen their anxiety
  - Tics
    - *Meta-analysis of controlled trials found that the risk of new-onset or worsening tics was similar in stimulant and placebo groups*
    - Monitoring of tics while on medications is recommended
  - Delayed Growth
    - *In 2014 Pediatrics, the official journal of the American Academy of Pediatrics published a longitudinal study by Harstad et al, concluded "ADHD treatment with stimulant medication is not associated with differences in adult height or significant changes in growth." (It is likely that these concerns stem from the fact that there are children who struggle with gaining weight due to lack of appetite adverse effect).*
    - Monitoring of growth for pediatric patients is recommended

Non-stimulant Drugs

- **Not** controlled substances; no abuse potential
  - Although stimulants are first line for ADHD, clinically non-stimulant medications are often trialed first

- Atomoxetine (Strattera)
  - MOA: Inhibits presynaptic reuptake of NE in the prefrontal cortex
  - Used for ADHD, especially if there is concern for addiction/abuse or exacerbating existing anxiety. *Clinical note – can still be used first even if no concern.*
  - Adverse effects - Appetite loss, fatigue, headache, cough, upset stomach, nausea

- Bupropion (Wellbutrin) – discussed above
  - See page 21

- Viloxazine (Qelbree)
  - See page 21

- Guanfacine ER (Intuniv) & Clonidine ER (Kapvay)
  - More commonly used for ADHD in **children**, but may also be trialed in adults
  - Most helpful with behavioral symptoms of ADHD

- MOA: **Alpha$_2$ agonists that mimic NE actions** in the prefrontal cortex via the stimulation of the Alpha$_2$A receptors
- Used for ADHD, generally reserved for behavioral especially if there is a concern for addiction/abuse
- Adverse effects – Sleepiness/sedation, fatigue, headache, dizziness, **hypotension** (possible rebound hypertension upon *discontinuation*), **arrhythmias**
- *Children treated with both a stimulant and the clonidine have shown significantly greater improvement in ADHD symptoms than those treated with a stimulant alone*

Alcoholism Treatments

- Naltrexone
  - **Reduces cravings**
  - MOA – **U-opioid antagonist** that reduces the pleasurable effects of a craving for alcohol. Helps both with alcohol cutback and with maintaining sobriety.
    - Cannot be combined with opioids (verify no opioids with **drug screen**)
    - Comes in long-acting injectable - Vivitrol
      - *Can be good for those with compliance issues with taking daily medications*
  - Routine lab monitoring – **LFTs**
  - Adverse effects include nausea, headaches, anxiety, and sedation
    - Black box warning – Severe liver disease so to not use in those with liver failure

- Acamprosate
  - Reduces cravings
  - MOA: **Glutamate receptor modulator**
  - Adverse effects include headache, diarrhea, flatulence, and nausea

- Disulfiram
  - Does not reduce or stop cravings
  - MOA: **Inhibits aldehyde dehydrogenase**, an enzyme that metabolize alcohol (blocks the breakdown of alcohol in the body that can cause patients on this medication to get sick upon drinking alcohol) – accumulation of acetaldehyde when alcohol is consumed
  - Acetaldehyde is toxic and induces nausea, vomiting, palpitations, hypotension

Considerations of comorbidities in choosing treatment

- Depression and history of sexual dysfunction
  - Consider bupropion/Wellbutrin or mirtazapine/Remeron

- Depression and focus/ADHD concerns
  - Consider bupropion/Wellbutrin

- Patients with history of HTN
  - Avoid SNRIs such as venlafaxine/Effexor
  - Avoid MAOIs due to tyramine induced hypertensive crisis

- Difficulty sleeping or poor appetite
  - Consider mirtazapine/Remeron

- Depression and poor appetite/low weight
  - Consider paroxetine due to weight gain side effect

- If history of cardiovascular disease
  - Caution with use of TCAs, SNRIs and MAOI

- If history of arrythmias
  - Avoid stimulants and medications that prolong QT interval (ex. Celexa, Lexapro)

- Patients with history of seizures
  - Avoid Bupropion due to decreased seizure threshold
    - Risk is thought to be lower with use of XR formulation
  - For patients with bulimia nervosa, vomiting is a factor that lowers seizure threshold. Avoid seizure threshold lowering medications in these patients as well.

- Patients with risk of poor compliance
  - Fluoxetine may be preferred due to long half-life limiting impact of missed doses
  - Long-acting injectable (LAI) helpful
    - Only available for certain medications (ex. Aristada, LAI for aripiprazole/Abilify; ex. Vivitrol, LAI for naltrexone)

- Patients with history of migraines
  - Lexapro has associated risk of general headaches which may trigger migraines

- Patients with chronic pain
  - Consider duloxetine/Cymbalta as it has been clinically shown to improve some pain symptoms

- Patients with IBS related abdominal pain
  - Consider amitriptyline

- Patients with risk of overdose (intentional or otherwise)
  - Avoid TCAs, avoid benzodiazepines

ADJUNCTIVE PSYCOTHERAPY

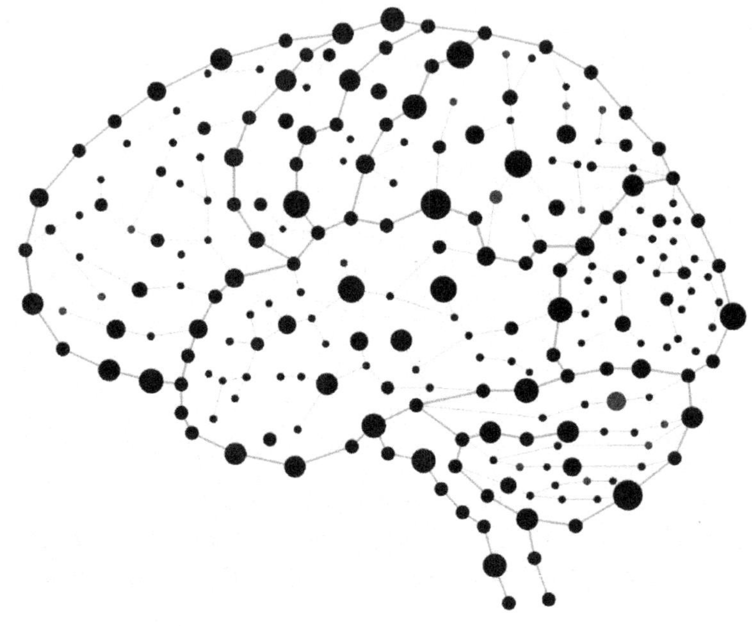

When treating psychiatric conditions, it is often imperative to combine pharmacological interventions with therapeutic support (Cuijpers et al., 2014). Therapy combined with medication, can help patients identify and address the root cause of their distress as well as provide adequate tools to manage symptoms long-term, provide a supportive and consistent relationship and improve self-esteem and interpersonal relatedness. It has also been demonstrated that therapy can improve adherence to medication, reduce relapse rates and improve overall well-being (Huhn et al., 2014).

There are a variety of evidence-based therapeutic modalities and techniques to treat mental health problems, each differing in their underlying premise and diagnostic focus. Among the most widely utilized therapy practices are cognitive behavioral therapy (CBT), dialectical behavior therapy (DBT) acceptance and commitment therapy (ACT), psychodynamic psychotherapy and mindfulness and somatic based therapies.

Cognitive Behavioral Therapy (CBT):

CBT is an empirically supported treatment for a vast array of psychiatric conditions. (Butler et al., 2006) It is based on the premise that psychological distress is often caused in part by irrational or maladaptive patterns of thought and behavior and that identifying, evaluating, and changing these patterns can lead to improved functioning and mental well-being. CBT also utilizes exposure and response prevention (ERP) to treat obsessive compulsive disorder and phobias. By exposing patients to their feared stimulus while systematically helping them habituate and regulate, they can learn to manage their anxiety during feared situations. CBT practitioners use these strategies to help patients reduce anxiety as well as improve coping skills, interpersonal relationships and general mood and functioning. One strength of CBT is its structured, directive approach and that it can be relatively short-term in duration, reducing issues of cost and accessibility. CBT has demonstrated effectiveness in treating major depression, generalized anxiety disorder, obsessive compulsive disorder, phobias, substance abuse disorders, marital problems, eating disorders, and psychosis (Hofmann, Asnaani, Vonk, Sawyer, & Fang, 2012).

Dialectical Behavior Therapy (DBT):

Originally developed by Marsha Linehan to treat borderline personality disorder, DBT is a psychoeducation-based therapy aimed at helping people learn to tolerate intense emotion, improve interpersonal functioning, reduce self-harming behaviors and suicidal ideation. DBT addresses four main areas of functioning including mindfulness, emotion regulation, distress tolerance, and interpersonal effectiveness. DBT also focuses on helping patients tolerate ambiguity and conflicting emotional experiences as part of the reality of life and relationships by teaching the concepts of the dialectic and walking the "middle path." DBT is effective in improving patients' ability to tolerate stress, reduce self-destructive behavior and engage in healthy and meaningful relationships. (Kliem, Kröger, & Kosfelder, 2010). DBT is often administered in a group setting and as part of an intensive treatment program with a family therapy component as well as access to an individual therapist who may provide 24-hour phone coaching support to help clients get through periods of intense distress. DBT has been effective in treating borderline personality disorder, reducing self-harm behaviors as well as treating depression, anxiety eating disorders and substance use disorders (Linehan, 2014).

Acceptance and Commitment Therapy (ACT):

ACT, proposed by Steven Hayes, is focused on enhancing psychological flexibility through mindfulness skills, acceptance strategies, and committed action in line with one's values. ACT utilizes tools and activities to explore a patient's thoughts, feelings, values, and goals to increase mindful awareness and acceptance of life as it is in the moment. ACT adheres to the idea that to live a fulfilling and meaningful life, one must accept negative or painful emotions and experiences as part of the human condition in its fulness. ACT is effective in treating anxiety and depression, chronic pain, obsessive compulsive disorder, eating disorders, substance use disorders and general life stress (A-Tjak et al., 2015).

Psychodynamic Psychotherapy (PDT)

PDT is derived from psychoanalysis, and both originate from the work of Sigmund Freud. PDT is an in-depth form of therapy that aims to help people better understand themselves through exploration of early life experiences, attachment style and relational patterns. PDT aims to alleviate psychological distress by addressing the origin and formation of psychological processes and personality structure through uncovering unconscious beliefs about the self, others and the world and exploring them in the context of a secure therapeutic relationship. Psychodynamic therapy is effective in treating a wide range of mental health symptoms including depression, anxiety, panic, and stress-related physical ailments and has demonstrated long lasting positive effects on well-being that increase over time (Shedler 2010).

Somatic and Mindfulness Based Interventions:

Somatic or body-oriented treatments are based on the premise that the mind and body of an individual are interconnected and must both be tended to for psychological well-being. Somatic Experiencing (SE), developed by Peter Levine, and Sensorimotor Psychotherapy, pioneered by Pat Ogden, are two prominent somatic approaches widely used in trauma treatment. Somatic therapies utilize tools to increase awareness of bodily sensations and look to the body as a guide to understanding and treating emotional distress and trauma. In addition, somatic therapies work to ground people mindfully in the present, reduce stress held in the body and releasee emotional tension by addressing the physiological aspects of trauma response, promoting a body-mind integration, and improving an individuals' capacity for self-regulation and emotional resilience (Parker, Doctor, and Selvam 2008).

Art Therapy (AT):

AT is a form of creative therapy founded on the belief that self-expression through artistic creation has therapeutic value. AT is used to improve cognitive and sensory-motor functions, foster self-esteem, and self-awareness, cultivate emotional resilience, promote insight, enhance social skills, reduce, and resolve conflicts and distress, and advance societal and ecological change (AATA, 2017). AT is utilized in the treatment of a wide range of mental health symptoms including stress, anxiety, depression, trauma, grief, personality disorders, physical illness, and disabilities. May be particularly useful in those with limited verbal/expressive ability, and those with dementia. Other creative therapies include dance movement therapy, drama therapy, music therapy and poetry therapy.

Conclusion:

Psychotherapy plays a crucial role as an adjunct to pharmacological treatment by offering a holistic, collaborative, and integrative approach to the treatment of mental illness. By combining the biochemical utility of medication with the work of evidence-based psychotherapy, clinicians can optimize treatment outcomes, reduce relapse, and improve overall patient well-being and life satisfaction.

DEPRESSIVE & ANXIETY RELATED DISORDERS

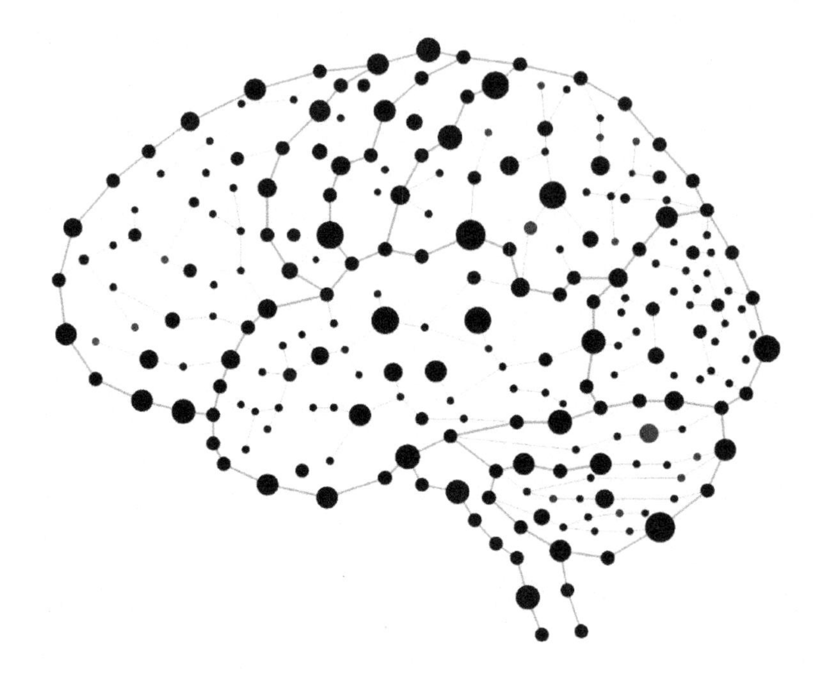

Major Depressive Disorder

Summary: Feeling down/disinterested most days due to environmental/genetic factors
S/S: Cognitive and psychomotor dysfunction that interfere with daily activities
Dx: Meet DSM 5 Criteria Symptoms last at least 2 weeks; PHQ-9 score of >5
Tx: Psychotherapy and SSRI are first line treatments

2nd line – Pathophysiology:

- Genetic → Thought to be hereditary in nature as it is **MC in first degree relatives of depressed parents**. Neurotransmitter dysfunction such as **abnormal regulation of catecholamines** (particularly norepinephrine), glutamines, serotonin, and cholinergic molecules; MTHFR gene is a common abnormality that can contribute to lack of neurotransmitters, B12/folic acid deficiencies can also contribute
    - Consider neuroendocrine function as a potential cause. Low levels of growth hormone or a hypo functioning pituitary gland may be a cause
- Environmental factors → Psychosocial factors such as **major life stressors** (loss, unemployment, separation) that may precede episodes of depression. May be secondary to a chronic medical illness. May occur without any preceding stressor as well.
- Some drugs may cause depression → corticosteroids, BB, interferon, amphetamines, alcohol, etc.
- Risk factors – suicide risk, F>M, **20s-30s** in age, exposure to daily stress, thyroid dysfunction, etc.
- Patients with depression are **more likely to abuse drugs/alcohol**

Clinical Manifestations:

- Grief is different than depression. Grief is negative feelings that occur in waves and are tied to a specific thought/event, and resolve when circumstances improve
- **Cognitive and psychomotor dysfunction that interferes with daily life** → Poor concentration, fatigue, low libido, trouble sleeping
- Various manifestations may occur during depressive episodes
    - <u>Anxious</u> – Patients feel tense and restless with difficulty concentrating, constant worrying
    - <u>Mixed</u> – Patients have ≥3 manic or hypomanic symptoms (elevated mood, flight of ideas)
        - Increased risk to develop bipolar disorder
    - <u>Melancholic</u> – Severe anhedonia that doesn't respond to positive stimuli

- Atypical – Mood improves with positive events with ≥2 of the following: overreact to criticism, feelings of a "paralysis", weight gain, increased appetite, hypersomnia
- Psychotic – Associated with delusions or hallucinations
- Catatonic – Severe psychomotor retardation that results in engaging in purposeless activity

- **Seasonal Affective Disorder** (SAD) – a type of depression but occurs during particular seasons of the year. Commonly winter months/months with less light, however can be any season (ex. in desert/hot climates summer months can be more common for SAD due to that season being the time where it is harder to leave the home).

- **MTHFR gene** – if pt has this genetic mutation a primary symptom is medication-resistant mood disorders, ex. depression non-responsive to SSRIs/psychotropic medications (often fail multiple psych meds/SSRIs due to lack of neurotransmitters secondary to gene abnormality)
    - Treated with L-Methyl Folate (supplement)

Diagnosis:

- Physical exam – tearful, avoid eye contact, lack facial expressions, slow or little body movement, etc.
- DSM-5 → **Must exist for at least 2 weeks and cause impairment in day-to-day life**
    - **Loss of interest/pleasure (anhedonia),** withdrawal from activities, guilt, etc.
    - ≥5 depressive symptoms: **depressed mood, anhedonia** (lack of interest/pleasure), weight loss/gain, insomnia or hypersomnia, fatigue, feelings of worthlessness/guilt, decreased ability to concentrate, psychomotor agitation/retardation (excessive movement/less movement than usual), SI
    - Not attributable to another substance or medical condition →R/o anemia, thyroid dysfunction (TSH, T4, Iron/TIBC/Ferritin/CBC H&H), folic acid/B12/vitamin D deficiencies
    - Recurrent thoughts of death or suicide
- Genetic testing for MTHFR gene (not required for MDD diagnosis but could be a contributing factor)
- PHQ-9 scale most used - Patient health questionnaire that assesses patients for depression. Commonly used in outpatient settings to screen for depression. Scored on scale of 0 through 27

Treatment:

- PHQ-9 score of 5-9 (Mild depression) – watchful waiting; psychotherapy may be used
- PHQ-9 score 10-14 (Moderate depression) - **psychotherapy** is 1st line
- PHQ-9 score of 15-19 (Moderately severe depression) – psychotherapy +/- SSRI
- PHQ-9 score of 20-27 (Severe depression) – psychotherapy + SSRI +/- ECT
    - All treatment should be individualized, and PHQ-9 scores should not be the sole determinant for how one chooses a treatment protocol
    - Recheck PHQ-9 at subsequent visits to assess treatment efficacy.
    - MTHFR gene mutation treated with L-Methyl Folate (supplement)
    - Treatment resistant depression (continued s/s despite at least 2 med trials with adequate dose and duration) option examples commonly used include cariprazine/Vraylar, aripiprazole/abilify, lithium, ketamine, spravato, TMS (transcranial magnetic stimulation, VNS (vagus nerve stimulation), etc.

Persistent Depressive Disorder (Dysthymia)

Summary: Long standing depression, a/w other mental health disorders and substance use
S/S: Feeling down most of the day most days
Dx: Symptoms last at least 2 years
Tx: Psychotherapy and SSRIs are first line

Pathophysiology:

- Think of this as MDD that lasts at least 2 years
- Symptoms begin during adolescence
- Risk factors: Family history**, substance use, personality disorder, anxiety disorder**
- Patho is the same as MDD (above)

Clinical Manifestations:

- Patients remain gloomy, pessimistic, introverted, lethargic, hypercritical of themselves **most days**

Diagnosis:

- DSM-5 – Depressed mood for **most of the day on most days for ≥2 years** with ≥ 2 of the following:
    - Poor appetite or overeating, insomnia or hypersomnia, fatigue, low self-esteem, poor concentration/difficulty making decisions, hopelessness

Treatment:

- 1st line - **Psychotherapy**
- 1st line pharmacological treatment - **SSRI**
- 2nd line options - SNRI, NRI, NDRI, atypical antidepressants, TCA, MAOI
- Refractory, pregnant, elderly → ECT and other interventional approaches

Suicidal/Homicidal Behaviors

Summary: Intent to self-harm or harm others with prior attempt being the biggest risk factor
S/S: MC method for suicide is drug ingestion; MC method for homicide is guns
Dx: Can use PHQ-9 scale to assess for suicidal ideation and f/u with a suicide severity scale
Tx: Admission likely; antipsychotics used in the acute setting

Pathophysiology:

- Suicidal ideation - Planning, considering, and/or thinking about suicide
- Attempted - **Nonfatal, self-directed act intended to cause death** that may or may not result in injury
- Non-suicidal self-injury - Self-inflicted pain or damage w/o intention of death
- Homicidal - Patient poses a risk to others, w/ intent to cause harm that results in death
- Risk factors - **Ages 45-64**, depression, mental health disorder, **military/veteran**, **transgender**, **alcohol/substance abuse**, men use more aggressive means, **prior suicide attempts** (BIGGEST RF), trauma in childhood, unemployment, family history
    - Men over the age of 50 are more likely to complete a suicide because of their tendency to attempt suicide with more violent means, particularly guns. On the other hand, women make more attempts but are less likely to complete a suicide
- Individuals hospitalized for depression have a lifetime suicide risk of 10-15%

Clinical Manifestations:

- Method - **Drug ingestion is MC method** (MC drug for intentional drug overdose is benzodiazepines – avoid these in patients with this history), violent methods uncommon; other methods include hanging, jumping from height, drowning, cutting, driving over a cliff
    - *Editor's note – be aware of medications prescribed that are lethal in overdose and intentionally provide less than that amount in one rx*
- In homicide, **shootings** are the MC method

Diagnosis:

- Clinical diagnosis
    - Different scales are used to assess severity. Start with a **PHQ-9** and if suicidal ideations present, complete a more specific scale such as the Columbia-Suicide Severity Rating Scale

Treatment:

- Clinicians must intervene and **transport patients to a secure environment. Patient is not to be left alone.** If outpatient call 911
- Patients may need to be **involuntarily committed or restrained**
  - Danger to self-prompts admission
    - Failure to attend to basic needs, self-harm, suicide attempt
  - Danger to others which prompts admission
    - Expressing homicidal intent, harming others
- Treatment options include **antipsychotics** (dopamine-receptor antagonists MC used), **lithium** (narrow therapeutic window and lethal in overdose so monitor closely), and ECT for acutely suicidal patients. **Psychotherapy** is used as an adjunct. Follow up closely.

Documentation shorthand:
S/H/I/I/P = suicidal homicidal ideation intent or plan
DTS/DTO = danger to self/danger to others

Generalized Anxiety Disorder

Summary: Constant worrying about anything and everything MC in F < 30 y/o
S/S: Worrying fluctuates and worsens with stress; worry about ALL aspects of life
Dx: DSM 5- Can't control worries for ≥6 months along with anxiety-like sx
Tx: Psychotherapy; SSRI is 1st line for pharm treatment

Pathophysiology:

- Risk factors – **Females** MC, under age 30 (develops during childhood), AA race, other mental health disorders (depression, panic disorder, substance abuse disorder), family history
- Thought to be hereditary
- Patho – Neurotransmitter disturbances in frontal lobe particularly **dopamine, NE, and serotonin imbalances** lead to the symptoms of anxiety

Clinical Manifestations:

- **Patients worry about everything** such as work, family, money, safety, responsibilities, tasks, etc.
- Clinical course fluctuates and always worsens with increased stress

Diagnosis:

- DSM-5 – Patients have difficulty controlling their worries for **≥6 months** with 3 of the following:
- Restlessness, fatigue, difficulty concentrating, muscle tension, irritability, and trouble sleeping
- Use the **GAD-7 questionnaire**:
  - Scores: 0-5 = None
  - 6-10 = Mild
  - 11-15 = Moderate
  - 16-21 = Severe

Treatment:

- Psychotherapy such as cognitive behavioral therapy (CBT) to learn relaxation and biofeedback
- Long term 1st line treatment – **SSRI**
  - 2nd line is SNRI
- Non-benzo anxiolytic that can be effective - buspirone (Buspar)
- For short term relief for acute, stressful episodic situations (ex. airplane flight or MRI scan) → short-acting benzodiazepine prn short term use; (prn use of propranolol or hydroxyzine is also common)

Panic Disorder

Summary: Repeated panic attacks w/ fear future attacks may occur due to sympathetic activity
S/S: Attacks last 5-20 min and are associated w/ increased sympathetic symptoms
Dx: ≥1 mo of persistent worrying about having an attack + 4 of 13 sx as per DSM
Tx: SSRIs are 1st line

Pathophysiology:

- Increased catecholamine surge triggered by the **SNS** due to fear
- Panic attacks: **Acute onset of a brief period of anxiety or fear with somatic/cognitive sx**
- Panic disorder – Repeated panic attacks with the fear that future attacks may occur
- Risk factors – **Females** affected twice as much as men, onset in mid 20s, stressful life situations

Clinical Manifestations:

- Attacks **peak within 10 minutes and last 5-20 minutes**
- Sometimes, symptoms are so severe, patients end up in the emergency room
- Panic disorder is defined by patients having the fear of having future attacks and it begins to impact their day-to-day life

Diagnosis:

- Recurrent, unexpected panic/anxiety attacks with fear about having another one that lasts for ≥ 1 month
- Patients must have **4 of the following 13 symptoms (increased sympathetic symptoms):**
  - Cognitive – fear of dying, fear of losing control, feelings of unreality/depersonalization
  - Somatic – chest pain, dizziness, choking feeling flushing/chills, nausea/abdominal pain, numbness/tingling, palpitations/tachycardia, shortness of breath, sweating, shaking/trembling
- Symptoms are not explained by any other disorder/condition
- DSM-5 – **For ≥ 1 month,** ≥ 1 attack has been followed by one of the following
  - **Persistent worrying** about having another panic attack or worrying about their consequences
  - Poor behavioral response to panic attacks such as **avoiding certain situations**

Treatment:

- 1st line – **SSRI**

        - Typically, medication should be continued for at least 1 year to prevent reoccurrence of symptoms
    - 2nd line – SNRI
    - For acute relief – propranolol and hydroxyzine commonly used; short term use of short acting benzodiazepines prn *(but ideally want to treat pt's baseline such as with SSRI so their panic threshold is reduced and they don't reach a panic attack to begin with; as opposed to just needing to abort them)*
    - Symptomatic relief - Beta Blockers help to lower heart rate and blood pressure, propranolol often as prn
    - Psychotherapy - **CBT** where they are taught how to think and modify their behavior

Editor's note – As anxiety is often worsened by the feeling that one is not in control, it may be helpful to explain just how normal anxiety is. In my practice I explain to patients that all people are the product of anxious ancestors. "Our ancestors hid in caves, while others went out and pet the lions. Those others, had no descendants. Anxiety is a survival mechanism, and it's only when it impedes and impacts your quality of life that it becomes a medical condition in need of a treatment". When discussing the use of SSRIs, I emphasize that it prevents them from reaching that panic threshold as easily or quickly. When discussing the use of prn medications, I describe it as an abortive, or in the example, a parachute. "When you feel like you are falling from 35,000 feet it's appropriate to deploy a parachute, but you shouldn't be walking around all day dragging a parachute behind you. Furthermore, just knowing you own the parachute is often enough to keep your panic at bay".

Post-Traumatic Stress Disorder (PTSD)

Summary: Recurring, intrusive thoughts "reliving" a traumatic event in thought
S/S: Intrusive thoughts of the trauma and avoidance of triggering stimuli
Dx: Sx of intrusion/avoidance, altered arousal, negative effect on mood for ≥1mo
Tx: Psychotherapy 1st line; SSRI commonly used; for nightmares -Prazosin

Pathophysiology:

- **Recurring, intrusive thoughts where one "re-lives" a traumatic event in their head**
- Patients may experience depersonalization or derealization
- Screening guidelines for military personnel - First visit and when needed, 60 days pre-deployment, 30 days post deployment, 3-6-month post deployment, annually
- Risk factors – **Military/veteran**, female gender, lack of family/social support, genetics (family history), low socioeconomic/ education status, **childhood trauma**, **sexual assault** (MC cause in females)

Clinical Manifestations:

- Negative alterations in cognition, mood (feeling emotionally numb), arousal and reactivity
- MC sx – unwanted thoughts, replaying memories of trauma occurring. +/- **nightmares,** <u>intrusive thoughts and avoidance must be present</u>
- Onset of symptoms begin to develop ≥6 months from the trauma
- **Acute stress disorder** – Occurs 3 days after the trauma but lasts **≤1 month**

Diagnosis:

- DSM-5 – Patients must be exposed to a traumatic event and have **symptoms from each of the main categories below for ≥1 month**. Must cause significant distress w/o obvious cause
    - **Intrusion symptoms** (Need ≥1 to meet diagnostic criteria)
        - Recurrent, intrusive, involuntary, disturbing memories
        - Nightmares of the event
        - Having flashbacks of the event and losing awareness in the present
        - Feeling intense psychological distress when reminded by the event
    - **Avoidance symptoms** (Need ≥1 to meet diagnostic criteria)
        - Avoid thoughts, feelings, memories associated with the event
        - Avoid activities, conversations, people, places that trigger memories of the event

- **Negative effects on cognition and mood** (Need ≥ 2 to meet diagnostic criteria)
    - Memory loss of significant parts of the event - Dissociative amnesia
    - Persistent and extreme negative beliefs/expectations about oneself or others
    - Persistent disorders thoughts about the trauma that lead to self-blame
    - Anhedonia
    - Feeling detached from others
    - Inability to experience positive emotions
- **Altered arousal/reactivity** (Need ≥ 2 to meet diagnostic criteria)
    - Difficulty sleeping
    - Irritability, an/ger, reckless or self-destructive behavior
    - Problems concentrating
    - Increased startle response
    - Hypervigilance

Treatment:

- 1st line – **Psychotherapy** (exposure therapy is often used)
- 1st linc pharmacological treatment – **SSRIs** (mainly sertraline, fluoxetine, escitalopram)
- For **nightmares** – **Prazosin** (alpha-blocker antihypertensive so monitor BP)
- Benzodiazepines are contraindicated for PTSD (often worsen sx severity and prognosis)
- Newer emerging treatments such as ketamine/mdma therapy

Specific Phobia

Summary: Unreasonable, intense fear of a specific object or situation that persists
S/S: Patients recognize that they overreact and that their fear is unreasonable
Dx: DSM 5 Marked fear or anxiety about specific object or situation for ≥ 6 mo
Tx: Exposure therapy

Pathophysiology:

- Defined as an **unreasonable, intense, overreaction of fear of a specific object or situation that persists**
- Commonly begins in childhood around age 12; May decrease in severity with age
- Risk factors –female gender, other psychiatric disorder
- The **most common of all the anxiety disorders** with MC phobias being related to animals (zoophobia), heights (acrophobia), confined places (claustrophobia), blood (hemophobia)

Clinical Manifestations:

- Symptoms depend on type of phobia (i.e. those with hemophobia may faint due to the vasovagal s/s)

Diagnosis:

- DSM-5 – Marked fear or anxiety about specific object or situation that lasts **for ≥ 6 months** that is not explained by another disorder plus all the following:
  - Situation provokes immediate fear/anxiety
  - Patients actively avoid it or endure with intense fear
  - Impairs function and interferes with day-to-day activities
  - **Fear/anxiety is out of proportion to actual danger**

Treatment:

- Drugs not effective – **Exposure therapy** is the best treatment
  - Through habituation, the anxiety surrounding a certain object/situation is relieved over time
- Propranolol (beta blocker) often used (hydroxyzine also common), or if refractory benzodiazepines short term prn to manage acute s/s

Social Phobia

Summary: Fear of embarrassment due to scrutiny/failure to meet expectations
S/S: Fear/anxiety related to being exposed to social situations
Dx: ≥6 mo marked fear/anxiety about social situations when exposed to scrutiny
Tx: Exposure therapy with CBT; SSRIs

Pathophysiology:

- Fear is centered around being embarrassed/humiliated due to scrutiny of others or failure to meet expectations (**public speaking is the MC type)**
- Risk factors – males and females equally affected, age ≤25, substance use

Clinical Manifestations:

- **Fear/anxiety related to being exposed to social situations**
- Patients avoid these situations or endure them with intense symptoms of anxiety

Diagnosis:

- DSM-5 – **Marked fear/anxiety about social situations** when exposed to scrutiny for ≥6 months plus:
  - Fears they will show anxiety symptoms and be negatively evaluated
  - **Avoid or endure social situations** with intense fear or anxiety
  - Fear/anxiety is **out of proportion** to actual threat and are not explained by another disorder
  - Symptoms cause distress/impair social/occupational functioning

Treatment:

- **Exposure therapy** with CBT is 1st line
- **SSRIs** are often used and effective
- Propranolol (beta blocker) often used (hydroxyzine also common), or if refractory benzodiazepines short term prn to manage acute s/s

Obsessive Compulsive Disorder

Summary: Patients have obsessions causing anxiety relieved by compulsions
S/S: Obsessions Recurrent, intrusive thoughts; Compulsions Repetitive behaviors
Dx: Time consuming (≥1 hour/day) obsessions/compulsions causing impairment
Tx: Cognitive/ritual prevention therapy; SSRI 1st line

Pathophysiology:
- **Obsessions create anxiety and are relieved by compulsive rituals**
- More common in females than males with age of onset in early 20s (some cases begin by age 14)
- Etiology is unknown but is thought to be due to a lack of serotonin
- High likelihood of co-existing mental health disorders

Clinical Manifestations:
- **Obsessions** - Recurrent, persistent thoughts that are intrusive and unwanted and cause anxiety or stress
- **Compulsions** - Repetitive behaviors or mental acts to try to relieve anxiety (**handwashing MC**, checking, counting, ordering)

Diagnosis:
- Clinical diagnosis - Rule out any other potential causes
- Time consuming obsessions or compulsions causes **significant distress or impairment**
  - **Lasting ≥1 hour/day** is considered time-consuming per DSM-5
- Yale Brown Obsessive Compulsive Scale can be used to aid diagnosis/track improvement

Treatment:
- **Cognitive therapy** along with exposure/ritual prevention therapy (for desensitization)
- **High doses of SSRIs** are 1st line for pharmaceutical treatment
  - Ex.) Fluvoxamine (Luvox); fluoxetine (Prozac), sertraline (Zoloft)
  - OCD sx can take up to 16 weeks to respond
  - OCD typically necessitates higher doses of SSRI than mood/anxiety/depression symptoms
  - Second generation/atypical antipsychotics (ex. aripiprazole) are often used if needed after SSRIs; less commonly clomipramine (TCA) is sometimes used
    - Supplement N-acetyl cystine has been shown to be helpful

BIPOLAR DISORDERS

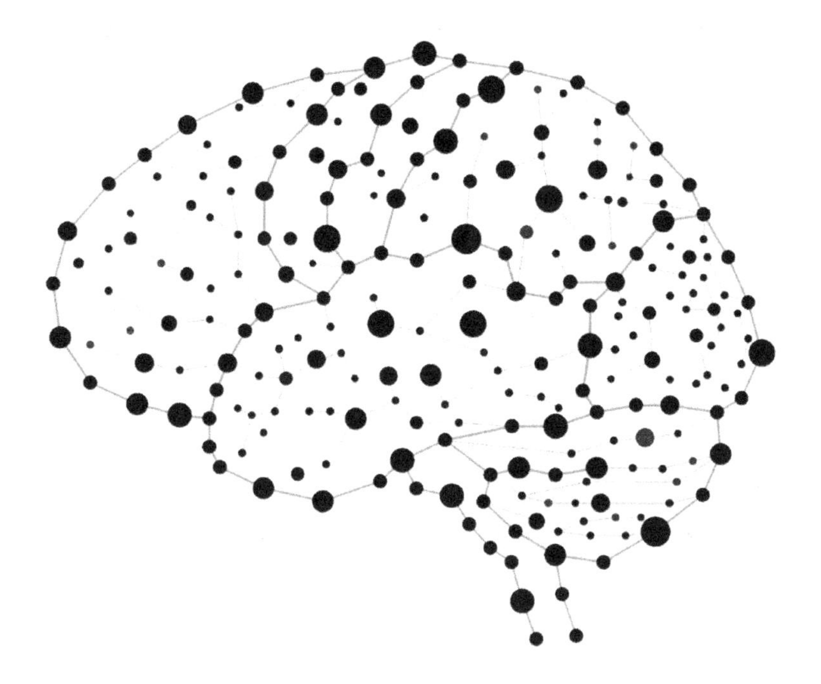

Bipolar Disorders (Type 1, 2, and Cyclothymia)

Summary: Alternating mania, hypomania, normal mood, and/or depression
S/S: Manic sx (elevated mood); Hypomanic sx (less extreme than mania)
Dx: BP I ≥7 days w/ ≥ 3 manic s/s or hospitalization/psychotic features.
BP II ≥4 days depression w/ ≥1 hypomanic episode
Tx: Mood stabilizers Lithium, anticonvulsants SgAs

Pathophysiology:

- Bipolar disorders: Associated with alternating periods of mania, depression, and normal mood
- Etiology is unknown but it is thought to be hereditary
    - Genetics
    - Dysregulation of serotonin, norepinephrine, and dopamine are involved
    - Psychosocial factors play a role
    - Cocaine/amphetamines, phencyclidines, antidepressants, enviro toxins worsen sx
- Thyroid disorders can cause similar symptoms, rule these out first (TSH/T4)
- Patients have a higher likelihood of attempting suicide (15 times greater than the population)
- Risk factors – family member with bipolar disorder, F>M, symptoms usually begin mid-adolescence through mid 20s, rare in children

Clinical Manifestations:

- Depression and at least one episode of mania or hypomania in lifetime
- Patients may or may not lack insight
- Rapid-cycling → presence of ≥4 mood episodes in 1yr of manic, hypomania, or depression
- Mania/hypomanic episodes include a distinct period of **persistently and abnormally elevated mood** with **≥3 manic symptoms** (or hyperirritable mood with greater than 4 manic sx)
    - **Mania** = **≥1 week** of manic symptoms with marked impairment in functioning, *or any length of manic episode that includes psychotic features OR necessitates hospitalization*
    - **Hypomania** (less extreme variant of mania) = **≥4 days** (but less than 7 days) of manic symptoms *(does not include psychotic features or require hospitalization),* episode not severe enough to cause marked impairment in functioning
- Manic symptoms:
    - Grandiosity/inflated self-esteem
    - Decreased need for sleep
    - Flight of ideas/racing thoughts
    - Rapid/excessive speech (more talkative than usual)

- Easily distractible
- Increased goal directed activity, increased interest in sex, psychomotor agitation
- Dangerous/rash decisions (ex. excessive/unrestrained spending, gambling

Diagnosis:

- DSM-5 – Rule out organic causers (ex. thyroid disease, drug use/abuse)
    - Bipolar I: At least one episode of **mania** in lifetime, with ≥3 manic symptoms (see list above), often also has major depressive episodes (during at least a 2-week period)
    - Bipolar II: At least one episode of **hypomania** (without mania) in lifetime with ≥3 manic symptoms (see list above) + at least one **major depressive episode** required (during at least a 2-week period)
    - Cyclothymia: ≥2 years for adults (1 year for kids) of chronic mood disturbance with periods of depressive episodes and hypomanic episodes *without ever meeting criteria* for mania, hypomania, or MDD

Treatment:

- Psychotherapy always used as an adjunct
- **Mood stabilizers** → lithium, anticonvulsants (lamotrigine, valproate, carbamazepine)
- 2nd generation antipsychotics (more common for bipolar type 1 and acute mania)

    Clinical note – if mania is present, 2nd gen antipsychotics are often preferred to treat acute mania; anticonvulsants are typically maintenance medications and may not be as effective at reducing acute mania

SCHIZOPHRENIA AND RELATED DISORDERS

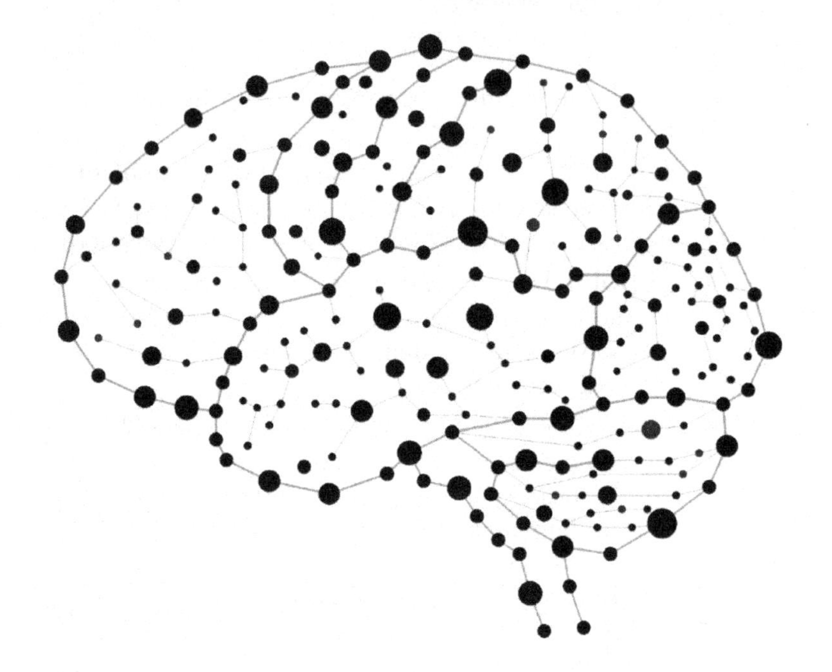

Schizophrenia (and related disorders)

Summary: Imbalances of dopamine lead to psychosis which impairs function
S/S: Positive sx → hallucinations, delusions, disorganized speech; Negative sx → poor affect, anhedonia, asociality
Dx: ≥2 schizophrenia symptoms for ≥6 months that cause functional disturbances
Tx: Second-gen/atypical antipsychotics and psychotherapy are first line

Pathophysiology:
- Etiology – unknown; thought to be secondary to ventricular enlargement, cortical atrophy, and hippocampus thinning
    - Glutamate hypothesis – ventricular enlargement, brain injury or birth complications, serotonin increase, decreased GABA are responsible for both positive and negative symptoms
    - Imbalances of dopamine result in decreased frontal lobe activity which is the cause of the symptoms
- The term schizophrenia translates to "split mind"
- Risk factors – male, onset at age 25-30, unemployed, substance use, recent hospital discharge, unmarried, prenatal infections, trauma/neglect in childhood

Clinical Manifestations:
- Psychosis - loss of contact with reality
- **Positive symptoms** occur secondary to **INCREASED dopamine** in the mesolimbic area - hallucinations, delusions, disorganized speech, grossly disorganized/catatonia/abnormal motor behavior
    - **Delusions** – thought as true in one's mind despite evidence otherwise
        - Persecutory – believe they are being tormented, followed, tricked, watched; that others are out to harm them
            - Ex) thinks the government is after them
        - Referential – believe show/song/article are directed at them
        - Somatic – thinks bodily sensations/functions are abnormal
            - Ex) Patient thinks they have an unrealistic illness or ailment
        - Grandiose – false belief of how great one is, exceptional abilities/fame/wealth
            - Ex) Believes they are immortal
        - Erotomanic – thinking another is in love with them
            - Ex) President of the USA is in love with patient
        - Jealous

            - Ex) Believes their significant other is cheating on them
        - Nihilistic - that a catastrophe may occur or that life is doomed, belief of being dead
            - Ex) Patient believes they do not exist, or they have passed away
        - Thought withdrawal or insertion – believe others can read their minds or insertion that thoughts were put in their mind
    - **Hallucinations** – sensory perceptions not perceived by anyone else
        - Auditory – MC
            - Command hallucinations – auditory hallucinations that instruct the person to do something
        - Visual
        - Tactile
        - Gustatory
        - Olfactory
        - Gustatory
    - **Disorganized thinking/speech** - symptoms include
        - Thought disorders and bizarre behaviors
            - Ex) loose associations/derailment
            - Ex) Neologism - making up new words
            - Ex) Unintelligible mixture of words/phrases; rhyming words
    - Grossly disorganized/abnormal/catatonic motor behavior
        - Unpredictable agitation
        - Difficulties with ADLs
        - Catatonia (add-on specifier) – decreased reaction to the world around them. Can exhibit rigid/bizarre posture.
- **Negative symptoms** occur secondary to **DECREASED dopamine** in the mesocortical region
    - Blunted affect – poor eye contact and lack of facial expressiveness
    - Poverty of speech - Patient speaks little and gives very short replies implying inner emptiness
    - Anhedonia – lack of interest in activities and increased purposeless activity
    - Asociality – lack of interest in relationships
    - Apathy
- Phases
    - Prodromal phase – little to no symptoms
    - Advanced prodromal phase – subclinical symptoms emerge (irritability, unusual thoughts, etc.)
    - Early psychosis phase – active symptoms are at their worst

- Middle phase – episodic periods of symptoms with worsening function
- Late illness phase – illness pattern may become stable, worsen, or dissipate

Diagnosis:

- DSM-5 – Patients must have **2 or more of the following 5 options** for **≥ 6 months**. AT LEAST 1 must be #1-3. Symptoms must cause a disturbance in functioning and are not attributable to any obvious causes (*rule out medications/illicit drugs/other physical causes i.e. infection, etc.*)
  - **1) Delusions**
  - **2) Hallucinations** (auditory MC)
  - **3) Disorganized speech**
  - 4) Grossly disorganized/abnormal/catatonic motor behavior
  - 5) Negative symptoms
- Brain imaging is not necessary but if performed, reveals abnormalities
  - CT scan – ventricular enlargement, cortical atrophy, hippocampus thinning
  - PET scan – decreased frontal lobe activity

Related disorders:

- For all of below: are not attributable to any obvious causes (rule out medications/illicit drugs/other physical causes i.e., infection, etc.)

Brief psychotic disorder

- Occurs due to psychological stress. MC in women, those with low socioeconomic status, and those with a personal history of a personality disorder
- Diagnostic criteria: Presence of **1 or more** psychotic symptoms (delusions, hallucinations, disorganized speech, grossly abnormal motor/catatonic behavior; at least one sx must be one of the first three (delusions, hallucinations, disorganized speech) for **1 day to 1 month** with return prior level of functioning thereafter

Schizophreniform disorder

- The same as schizophrenia except symptoms last anywhere from 1 through 6 months
- Diagnostic criteria: Patients must have 2 or more of the 5 schizophrenia sx for 1-6 months. AT LEAST 1 must be #1-3 (delusions, hallucinations, disorganized speech)

Schizoaffective disorder

- MC in females
- Diagnostic criteria: **At least one major mood episode (major depression or mania)** concurrent with symptoms of schizophrenia

- + **Psychotic sx (delusions or hallucinations) lasting ≥2 weeks** in absence prominent mood symptoms (depression or mania)

Delusional disorder
- Persistent delusion can have little to no effect on one's ability to function
- Diagnostic criteria: Prescence of 1 or more delusions for ≥1 month
- Types of delusions – see above

Positive prognostic factors
- Associated w/ a good prognosis – acute onset, short prodrome, age of onset late 20s-30s, mood symptoms present, negative symptoms absent, female gender

Negative prognostic factors
- Associated with a poor prognosis – insidious onset, prodrome began in childhood, onset in early teenage years, absent mood symptoms, present negative symptoms, and male gender

Treatment:
- Atypical (2nd generation) antipsychotics 1st line, decrease dopamine and serotonin
    - Second generation antipsychotics have LESS EPS symptoms (although EPS sx are still possible)
    - Due to metabolic side effects, second generation antipsychotics require lab follow up such as CBC, CMP, LP, A1C, TSH, prolactin.
    - Long-acting injectable versions becoming more common which help with compliance (ex. aristada)
- Typical (1st generation) antipsychotics 2nd line, decrease dopamine
- **Typical antipsychotics work best to treat NEGATIVE symptoms** and **atypical antipsychotics are most effective in managing POSITIVE symptoms**
- Treatment for similar disorders:
    - Brief psychotic disorder – **self-limited** and typically does not require the use of antipsychotics
    - Schizophreniform disorder – treat the same as schizophrenia with antipsychotics
    - Delusional disorder – psychotherapy, as medications are not very effective
    - Schizoaffective disorder – treated the same as schizophrenia, second generation antipsychotics utilized. Paliperidone is commonly used.
        - Antidepressants are sometimes added as an adjunct

For refractory symptoms – ECT can be considered

SUBSTANCE ABUSE DISORDERS

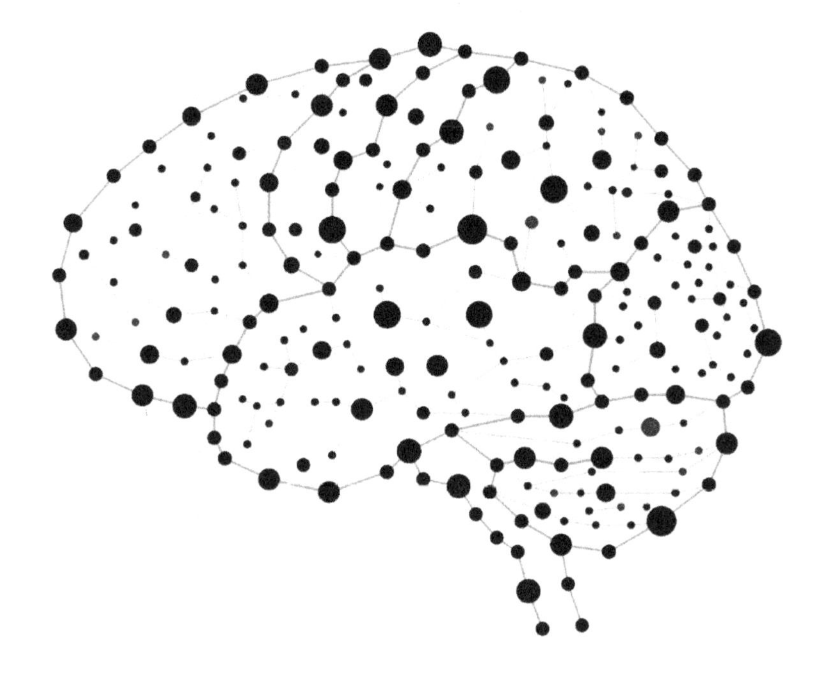

Alcohol Use Disorder / Withdrawal

Summary: Addiction to drinking EtOH leading to intoxication and/or withdrawal
S/S: AUD Intoxication and hepatic dysfunction; withdrawal, tremors, DTs
Dx: EtOH use disorder ≥2 symptoms in 12 months; Labs LFTs, GGT, BAC, CDT
Tx: Dependency – Naltrexone, disulfiram; Withdrawal – librium, glucose, vitamins; DT– benzo

- Ask patients how many "drinks" they have. A drink is equal to **12 ounces of beer, 8 ounces of malt liquor, 5 ounces of wine, or 1.3 ounces of liquor** (80 proof alcohol)
- MC abused substance
- Risk factors - occupations such as bartenders, tobacco users, gambling use disorder, mood/anxiety disorder, antisocial personality disorder, M>F, medical/surgical patients, broken home, unmarried, Native Americans, family history (may be genetic)
- Screening at annual visits for those ≥18 years old
  - **CAGE questionnaire (see table 1 on next page)**
  - **Positive w/ affirmative answer to 2 or more questions,** also positive if they affirm the need for an "eye opener" (a drink to start the day)

Table 1. CAGE Questionnaire

C	Have you felt the need to **C**ut down?
A	Have you felt **A**nnoyed when people suggest a drinking problem?
G	Have you felt **G**uilty about drinking too much?
E	Do you need an **E**ye opener in the morning?

Clinical Manifestations:

- At risk:
  - **MEN ≥ 4 drinks per day OR 14 drinks per week**
  - **WOMEN ≥3 drinks per day OR 7 drinks per week**
- Patients are often depressed, suicidal, homicidal
- Early symptoms of alcohol use disorder - Development of acne rosacea, palmar erythema, fatty infiltrates produce painless enlargement of liver, respiratory or other infections, unexplained bruises secondary to anemia, periods of amnesia, accidents (unexplained falls, driving concerns/DUI, arrest)
- Advanced symptoms of alcohol use disorder - Jaundice or ascites, testicular atrophy, gynecomastia, Dupuytren's contracture, psychosocial
- **Acute intoxication – drowsiness, psychomotor dysfunction, disinhibition, ataxia, nystagmus**

- Withdrawal symptoms
    - **Mild (begins 8 hrs – 3 days) – tremors, elevated vital signs, & anxiety**
    - **Moderate (24 – 36 hrs)** – **seizures,** autonomic instability
    - **Severe (24 – 72 hrs)** – **delirium tremens (DT)**, mental confusion, tremors, sensory hyperacuity, visual hallucinations, autonomic hyperactivity, diaphoresis, dehydration, & electrolyte imbalance
        - Delirium tremens is a medical emergency and life-threatening condition, 5-15% mortality if left untreated; may also be delayed more than a week with peak intensity at 4-5 days after last drink
- Complications include memory/recall problems
    - **Wernicke's Encephalopathy** – confusion, ataxia, and ophthalmoplegia that is reversible
    - **Korsakoff Syndrome** – anterograde and retrograde amnesia with confabulation
- Both severe alcohol intoxication and alcohol withdrawal can be fatal

Diagnosis:

- DSM-5 for Alcohol Use Disorder (AUD) – **≥2 symptoms within a 12-month period:**
    - Alcohol taken in large amounts or over longer period than intended
    - Persistent desire or unsuccessful attempt to cut down /control use
    - Great deal of time spent on activities necessary to get alcohol
    - Craving, or a strong desire/urge for alcohol
    - Recurrent use resulting in failure in other obligations (work, home, school)
    - Continued use despite having recurrent social and interpersonal problems
    - Important social, occupational, recreational activities are given up or reduced 2nd to alcohol use
    - Recurrent use in situations while physically hazardous
    - Alcohol use is continued despite knowledge of having a persistent physical/psychological problem caused by alcohol
    - **Tolerance** – having to drink more to feel the effects of the alcohol
- Labs for intoxication:
    - **Blood alcohol content** (BAC)
        - 20-50 mg/dL – mild sedation and slight decrease in fine motor conduction
        - 50-100 mg/dL – impaired judgement and more motor coordination deficits

        - 100-150 mg/dL – unsteady gait, nystagmus, slurred speech, memory impairment
        - 150-300 mg/dL – delirium and lethargy
    - **High LFTs** (often 1st test ordered)
    - Check electrolytes – low potassium and magnesium
    - High uric acid
    - High gamma-glutamyl transferase (GGT) – better test than LFTs for acute intoxication
    - **Carbohydrate-deficient transferrin (CDT)** – most definitive for chronic use as it detects if someone is a binge drinker or daily heavy drinker

Treatment:

- Alcohol use disorder/dependency
    - **Alcoholics Anonymous** is 1st line – self-help group and provides patients with non-drinking friends
    - **Naltrexone** (also comes in long-acting injectable – Vivitrol), **acamprosate**, **disulfiram**
- Wernicke's Encephalopathy and Korsakoff Syndrome – treatment for both includes **Thiamine IV** followed by **glucose**
- Supplement with vitamin B12, folic acid, thiamine, and glucose PRN
- Avoid medications that lower seizure threshold – bupropion, haloperidol, anticonvulsants, clonidine, beta blockers

- Withdrawal – mainstay **inpatient**
    - High dose **benzodiazepines** (lorazepam, oxazepam, temazepam)
    - **Librium** (chlordiazepoxide) if patients have ≥3 of the 7 symptoms
        - Systolic BP ≥160
        - Diastolic BP ≥100
        - HR ≥110
        - Temperature ≥ 38.3° C
        - Nausea
        - Vomiting
        - Tremor
    - **Thiamine**
    - **Folic acid**
    - Clonidine (alpha 2 agonist) – reduces symptoms of hypertension and tachycardia
    - For hallucinations – antipsychotics such as Haloperidol or Risperidone
    - **Delirium tremens** (DT) – diazepam/lorazepam
    - Seclusion and restraints as necessary
    - Adequate hydration and nutrition

Tobacco Use Disorder

Summary: Highly addictive due to nicotine, which leads to dependence in as little as 2 weeks
S/S: Increases heart rate, BP, respiratory rate, concentration, energy, sense of pleasure
Dx: Detailed history is crucial to council patients
Tx: OTC nicotine patches, gums, lozenges, etc.; Rx Wellbutrin or Chantix

Pathophysiology:

- Smoking prevalent in men, young adults, lesbian/gay/bisexual/transgender, disabled, education less than high school, people below poverty income level, those with psych disorders, alcohol/substance use, American Indian/Alaskan n7atives. It is less common in Hispanics and Asian women
- Wide variety of exposures - Cigars, pipes, e-cigs, vape devices, chewing tobacco, and passive exposure to smoke (in home, work)
- Patho →**Nicotine is highly addictive** (cravings can begin within days) → stimulates brain nicotinic receptors releasing dopamine and other neurotransmitters, which active the brain reward system during pleasurable activities in a manner like that of many addictive drugs.
- Psychologic and physical dependence can begin in as little as 2 weeks
- Chronic effects →**CAD, lung cancer, COPD**
- In exposed children →SIDS, asthma, otitis media, orofacial clefts (if exposed in home or in utero), low fetal birth weight

Clinical Manifestations:

- Nicotine **increases HR, BP, RR, increased energy/arousal, increased concentration, decreased tension/anxiety, sense of pleasure and reward, nausea in new users, decreased appetite**
- Toxicity can occur if ingested (like children eating cigarettes or gum)
  - Mild – N/V, h/a, weakness; symptoms resolve within 1-3 hours
  - Severe – cholinergic toxidrome with N/V, salivation, lacrimation, diarrhea, urination, fasciculations, muscle weakness, crampy abdominal pain, arrhythmias, hypotension, seizures, coma; can last 24 hours
- Withdrawal – **craving cigarettes**, difficulty concentrating, depression, anxiety, sleep disruptions, and weight gain

Diagnosis:

- Detailed history! Smoking within 30 min of waking indicates problematic use
- Prevention – prevent youth from smoking; 90% of smokers start before age 18

Treatment:

- Poisoning – supportive
    - Airway protection and ventilation if needed
    - Seizures – benzos
- Smoking cessation – therapy and counseling
    - **OTC nicotine patches, gums, lozenges, inhalers** are widely available
    - Bupropion (Zyban/Wellbutrin) – increase NE and dopamine
        - Do not use in patients with seizure disorder or eating disorder
    - Varenicline (Chantix) – partial agonist at the nicotinic acetylcholine receptor
        - Most effective

Take-Away Points for Overdose/Poisonings

Substance	Symptoms	Treatment
Alcohol	Tremors, seizures, DTs	High dose Benzo, Librium
Cocaine	Sympathetic activation	Supportive care → Benzos
Benzo	Respiratory distress	Flumazenil
Opioids	Resp depression, pupil constriction	Narcan

Cannabis Related Disorder

Summary: MC used illicit drug; Can be ingested, insufflated, vaporized, topical
S/S: Intoxication Lack of motivation, increased appetite, dry mouth, red eyes
Dx: Stays in urine for 1-3 days in infrequent users and up to a month in chronic/heavy users
Tx: Supportive care for withdrawal

Pathophysiology:

- Cannabis aka marijuana, pot, weed, etc
  - Active ingredients are cannabinoids (bind to cannabinoid receptors in the brain)→ Delta-9-tetrahydrocannabinol (THC) → **THC** is lipid soluble, so it takes time to be metabolized and excreted
- Gateway drug (highly controversial) → Leads to patients exploring other drugs
- Common in people with mental disorders and causes increased risk of schizophrenia
- Most used illicit drug but causes very little physical dependence → Legal in some states
- Can be **ingested, insufflated, vaporized, and applied topically** as a lotion or spray
- **Affects the hippocampus and causes cognitive impairment** if started in adolescence
- Prenatal marijuana use is associated with low fetal weight

Clinical Manifestations:

- Amotivational syndrome is associated with cannabis use
- Chronic use of THC can upregulate/exacerbate **anxiety**
- High-dose smokers → Pulmonary s/s → Wheezing, coughing, phlegm (not obstructive airway disease)
- Intoxication → Euphoria, serenity, increased thirst/appetite, improved confidence, heightened vigilance, red eyes, tachycardia, dry mouth, cough, memory deficits, time/color/spatial perception is altered
- Intoxication occurs within 10 – 30 minutes; half-life is about 50 hours
- **Cannabinoid hyperemesis syndrome** → Cyclic episodes of nausea and vomiting in chronic users
- **Cannabis induced psychosis** → fairly common manifestation (and the younger it occurs, the increased likelihood of psychotic symptoms persisting beyond the time of intoxication)
- Withdrawal (seen only w/heavy use) → Mild symptoms 12 hrs after last use that may last up to 7 days
  - Nausea, depression, insomnia, anorexia, irritability, anxiety

Diagnosis:

- **Urine is MC tested → Positive 1-3 days in infrequent users (≤2 times/week),** 7-21 days in moderate users, and up to 1 month in heavy users
- Saliva tests are positive for up to 24 hours after use; Hair test most sensitive and positive up to 90 days
- Blood tests only positive up to 3-4 hours

Treatment:

- **Supportive;** benzos/anxiolytics are sometimes used to help with anxiety and agitation
- **Cannabinoid hyperemesis syndrome** →IV fluids, antiemetics; hot showers have been shown to be helpful
- Behavioral therapy in outpatient drug treatment program

Inhalant Intoxication/Use Disorder

Summary: Intentional or unintentional exposure to volatile hydrocarbon toxic gas
S/S: Hypoxia, dizziness, incoordination, depressed reflexes, slurred speech, euphoria
Dx: Hx of exposure, psychological changes and physical symptoms correlating with exposure
Tx: Supportive care, maintain breathing/airway/circulation, abstinence

Pathophysiology:

- Inhalation/ aspiration of **hydrocarbon**-based inhalants like **gasoline, solvents, paints, glue,** and others that produce these toxic gases.
  - The higher the volatility (tendency of a liquid to become a gas) the higher the likelihood of intoxication
  - CNS effects due to that many hydrocarbons cross the blood-brain barrier, but these effects also be an indirect result from hypoxia or hypercarbia
  - Hydrocarbons are generally neurologic depressants
  - Hypoxia develops due to ventilation/perfusion mismatch
  - "Sudden sniffing death syndrome" → shortly after inhalation, usually when "excited" a surge of catecholamines, in conjunction with the hydrocarbons side effect of increased myocardium sensitization, increasing the risk of arrhythmias
- Common in underaged **youth** individuals as these substances are legal and have easier access
- Informally known as "huffing" or "bagging"
  - Substances put into a bag more likely to lead to hypercarbia
- 10% of 13–17-year-olds report using an inhalant at least once. Only 0.4% of 12–17-year-olds progress to inhalant use disorder.

Clinical Manifestations:

- Respiratory complaints, hypoxia, HA, cognitive impairment
- Pulmonary toxicity
  - Most common complaint is respiratory; coughing, hypoxia, increased work of breathing
  - Hydrocarbon pneumonitis can occur (the destruction of alveoli and capillary membranes) which can eventually lead to ARDS
- Cardiac toxicity
  - Arrhythmias -ventricular tach or v-fib
- CNS effects
  - Primary one = decreased level on consciousness
  - Initial s/s may be agitation, hallucinations, tremors
- GI effects

        - More common with ingestion as opposed to inhalation → burning sensation, abdominal pain, nausea/vomiting
- Intoxication occurs within 30 minutes, but could be delayed up to hours
- Cravings, tolerance, withdrawal often seen in inhalant use disorder
    - With prolonged exposure - rashes, chronic headaches, white matter degeneration, peripheral demyelination, peripheral neuropathy, or cognitive impairment

Diagnosis:

- Inhalant **intoxication** DSM-5 – Intended or unintended exposure to inhalant volatile hydrocarbons + behavioral/physiological effects (impaired judgement, belligerence, etc.) post-exposure, and **two** or more of these symptoms. Symptoms are not attributable to any obvious causes (rule out intoxication from another substance.
    - Dizziness
    - Nystagmus
    - Incoordination
    - Slurred speech
    - Unsteady gait
    - Lethargy
    - Depressed reflexes
    - Psychomotor retardation
    - Tremor
    - Generalized muscle weakness
    - Blurred vision or diplopia
    - Stupor or coma
    - Euphoria
- **Inhalant Use Disorder** DSM-5 – Problematic hydrocarbon-based inhalant use over time causing impairment/distress w/in 12-month period.
    - 2 of the following **w/in a 12-month period**:
        - Larger amounts or over a longer period than was intended
        - Unsuccessful efforts to stop or cut down use
        - Significant time obtaining/using/recovering the substance
        - Cravings
        - Use causes neglect of responsibilities (work/school/home)
        - Continued use despite problems caused by use
        - Important personal activities are stopped/lessened due to use
        - Recurrent use in physically dangerous situations
        - Continued use despite knowledge of having a problem with the substance
        - Tolerance

Treatment:

- **Supportive** – control airway, brcathing, and circulation
- Significant exposure → administering supplemental oxygen
- Watch for changes on pulse oximetry or chest radiography at least 6 hrs

Cocaine Related Disorder

Summary: A sympathomimetic drug that enhances NE, dopamine, and serotonin Euphoria
S/S: Intoxication Pupillary dilation, weight loss, hallucinations, formication
Dx: Urine metabolite Benzoylecgonine is positive 48-72 hours after use
Tx: Supportive; benzos for agitation/seizures, IV Nitrates for HTN, cooling for hyperthermia

Pathophysiology:

- Cocaine is a **sympathomimetic drug that can be snorted or injected intravenously** which creates a sense of euphoria and **stimulates the CNS** →Enhances NE, dopamine, and serotonin activity
  - Block Na channels – local anesthetic, **vasoconstriction** causes sequala of life-threatening s/s
- Risk when taken with alcohol due to cardiotoxic metabolite cocaethylene

Clinical Manifestations:

- High doses – **schizophrenia like symptoms, seizures, stroke, aortic dissection, mesenteric ischemia, myocardial infarction, hypertension, hyperthermia, arrhythmia, rhabdomyolysis**
- Very short acting (**10-15 minutes**) so patients may repeatedly smoke it
- Intoxication – euphoria, pupillary dilation, hypervigilance, anxiety, N/V, irritability, weight loss, weakness, paranoia, hallucinations, **formication** (itchy skin as if bugs are crawling on patients)
- Overdose – respiratory depression, arrhythmias, MI, seizures, hemorrhage, hallucinations, agitation, delusions, impairment, **mydriasis, diaphoresis, palpitations**
- Withdrawal – dysphoria, increased appetite, anhedonia, vivid/unpleasant dreams, **depression, fatigue, sleep issues, difficulty concentrating, somnolence** (cocaine wash out syndrome)
- In pregnancy – increased risk of placental abruption and spontaneous abortion

Diagnosis:

- **Urine metabolite** – **benzoylecgonine is positive 48-72 hours after use**

Treatment:

- Overdose – supportive treatment since the metabolites are so short acting
  - **IV Benzodiazepine** for agitation, hypertension, seizures
  - IV nitrates for HTN

    - Avoid BB (allow continued alpha-adrenergic stimulation)
- Cooling techniques if hyperthermic

Opioid Related Disorder

Summary: Opioids bind to the μ receptor to produce an analgesic effect, High addictive risk
S/S: Withdrawal produces flu-like sx; Intoxication causes euphoria, sedation
Dx: + in urine for 2-7 days; Opioid use disorder ≥2 DSM 5 criteria for 12-months
Tx: Withdrawal – methadone; acute intoxication – naloxone (Narcan)

Pathophysiology:

- Opioids are natural, semisynthetic, or synthetic compounds such as morphine, heroin, hydrocodone, oxycodone, codeine, tramadol, meperidine that **bind to opioid receptors (μ) and have a high potential for addiction and ultimately abuse**
- Indications for use include analgesics, anesthetics, cough suppressants, antidiarrheals

Clinical Manifestations:

- **Withdrawal produces flu-like symptoms** – lacrimation, rhinorrhea, sweating, yawning, piloerection, hypertension, tachycardia, hot/cold flashes, abdominal cramp, diffuse diarrhea, nausea, vomiting, joint/muscle aches, seizures, anxiety, restlessness, irritability, insomnia, decreased appetite
- Intoxication causes **euphoria, constipation, sedation**
- Highest morbidity of psychiatric conditions due to overdoses

Diagnosis:

- Physical exam – pupil constriction, **respiratory depression**, bradycardia, hypotension, **biot breathing** (groups of quick shallow inspirations followed by regular/irregular periods of apnea)
- Opioid use disorder as per DSM-5 – **≥2 of the following over a 12-month period**:
    - Taking opioids in larger amounts or for a longer time than intended
    - Persistently desiring or unsuccessfully attempting to decrease opioid use
    - Spending a great deal of time obtaining, using, or recovering from opioids
    - Craving opioids
    - Failing repeatedly to meet obligations at work, home, or school because of opioids
    - Continuing to use opioids despite having recurrent social or interpersonal problems
    - Giving up important social, work, or recreational activities because of opioids
    - Using opioids in physically hazardous situations

    - Use opioids despite having a physical/mental disorder caused or worsened by opioids
    - Having tolerance to opioids (not a criterion when use is medically appropriate)
    - Having opioid withdrawal symptoms or taking opioids because of withdrawal
- Withdrawal symptoms begin between 6 to 24 hours of discontinuation
    - Can test urine, saliva, blood, hair – **positive in urine for 2-7 days**, saliva for 5 hours, blood for 6 hours, and hair up to 90 days

Treatment:

- Withdrawal – **Methadone** (synthetic opioid agonist) in an inpatient or outpatient setting
- Other medications for withdrawal:
    - Clonidine – Centrally acting to reduce the autonomic AE via alpha blockade
    - NSAIDS – For musculoskeletal related pain
    - **Dicyclomine (Bentyl)** – For diarrhea associated with withdrawal – reduces GI muscle spasms
- Opioid dependent treatment:
    - **Acute intoxication** – **Naloxone** (**Narcan**)
        - A competitive antagonist with the highest affinity for the μ receptor
    - **Methadone** maintenance therapy (can be used for short term)
    - **Suboxone (Buprenorphine/Naloxone)** - Generally used for maintenance and dependent states
        - Buprenorphine is a partial opioid agonist that binds μ receptors to produce analgesic effects
    - Be aware – relapses common; regular drug screens needed
- Sleep hygiene and rehab are often used as adjuncts to the above medical treatments

Benzodiazepine Related Disorder

Summary: Benzos increase GABA, an inhibitory neurotransmitter, that makes them addictive
S/S: Overdose → Respiratory distress/arrest; Withdrawal, agitation, ataxia
Dx: Urine test is MC; Shows up 4-7 days post use in chronic users
Tx: Flumazenil for overdose; Benzo taper for withdrawal

Pathophysiology:

- Benzos are used for withdrawal syndrome, short term for sleep disorders, anxiety disorders, panic attacks, multi-use in psychopharmacology (increases chloride influx into cells)
- Benzos **increase GABA** (primary inhibitory neurotransmitter), which creates a calming effect

Clinical Manifestations:

- Overdose – **respiratory distress/arrest** especially with alcohol, depression, labile mood
- Withdrawal (24 hrs-14 days) - Anxiety, nightmares, agitation, tachycardia, anorexia, noise sensitivity, blurred vision, paresthesia, seizures, muscle spasms, hyperpyrexia, insomnia, life threatening
    - Abrupt discontinuation/withdrawal of benzodiazepines can be fatal

Diagnosis:
Common

- Urine, blood, hair, saliva tests →**Urine** is MC; shows up 1 week post discontinuation in chronic users

Treatment:

- Overdose → respiratory support and restraints
    - **Flumazenil for acute reversal** (NOT used in withdrawal; reduces seizure threshold)
- Withdrawal → benzodiazepine taper, often swapped to diazepam
    - Tapering typically used longer acting benzodiazepines and is done slowly over a long-term periods as rapid discontinuation can cause withdrawal concerns (may take 48 hours to 2 weeks to develop withdrawal sx), depends on how long the patient has been using the medications; *taper off period can last months.*

POISONINGS & INTOXICATION

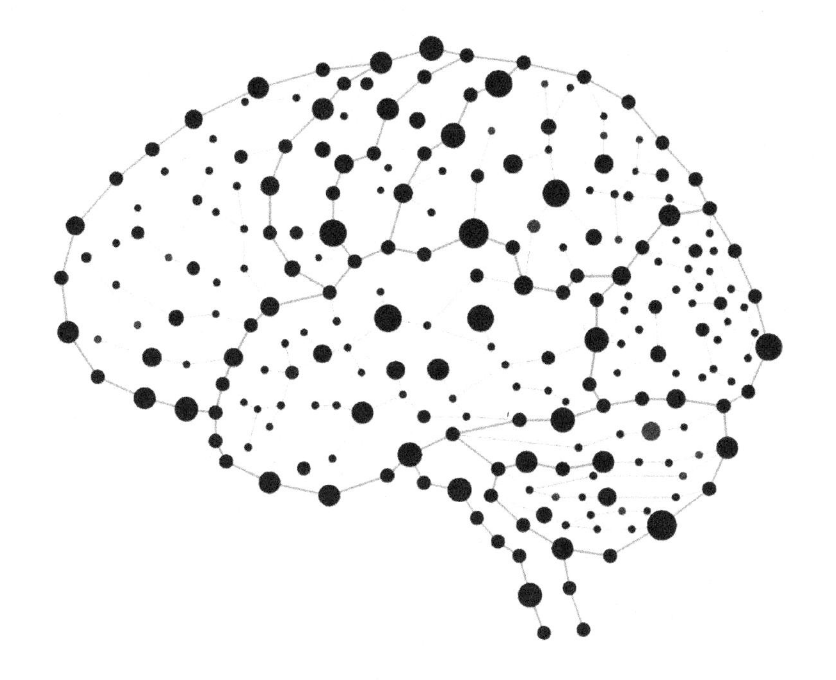

Hallucinogen Intoxication

Summary: Hallucinogens affect DA, SA, ACH, and GABA receptors. Unpredictable reactions
S/S: PCP – assaultive behavior; LSD – increased feeling of attachment to others
Dx: PCP – found in urine up to 2 weeks after last use and rotary nystagmus on PE
Tx: Supportive treatment

Pathophysiology:

- Diverse group of compounds, both synthetic and botanical: lysergic acid diethylamide (LSD), mescaline, methylenedioxymethamphetamine (MDMA; ecstasy), phencyclidine (PCP), psilocybin
  - LSD – taken orally with 30-60 min onset of action and effects up to 24 hours
  - Psilocybin – from several types of mushrooms consumed orally with effects lasting up to 6 hours.
    - In studies for refractory treatment resistant depression
  - Mescaline – from peyote cactus; taken orally with 30-90 min onset of action and 12 hr effect
- Affect several neurotransmitters: **dopamine, serotonin, anticholinergic, & GABA**
- **Cause unpredictable, idiosyncratic reactions**

Clinical Manifestations:

- Hallucinations, perceptual distortions, feeling of unreality, **synesthesia** (seeing sounds, hearing colors)
  - Psilocybin and mescaline are MC associated with hallucinations
- **Sympathomimetic** properties – tachycardia, HTN, seating, blurry vision, tremors, mydriasis
- PCP - Psychotic features with **assaultive behavior** *(very potent)*
- LSD - Intense feeling of attachments to others, high energy, serenity, **desire for sex**, visual hallucinations, blurred vision, mydriasis, sweating, palpitations

Diagnosis:

- Overdose – Medical emergency (hyperpyrexia, tachycardia, arrhythmias, stroke, dehydration, coma, seizures, death)
- PCP use -Look for agitation, disorientation, hallucination, delirium, vertical, horizontal, and **rotary nystagmus**, extraordinary physical strength
- Only PCP is included in routine urine drug screens and can be **positive for up to 2 weeks** after last use

        - Can also be tested via hair for up to 90 days, blood for up to 24 hrs, and saliva for up to 48 hrs

Treatment:

- o Diazepam for agitation
- o Haloperidol/ Risperidone for behavioral disturbances

Anticholinergic Intoxication

Summary: Inhibition of muscarinic receptor → life threatening sx if abused
S/S: Flushing, dry skin/MM, fever, mydriasis, tachycardia, ileus, urinary retention
Dx: Assess for arrhythmias, other drugs, cultures if febrile, ABG for acid/base
Tx: Physostigmine salicylate is a cholinesterase inhibitor, shown to reduce delirium

Pathophysiology:

- Inhibition of cholinergic neurotransmission at **muscarinic receptor sites in the central and peripheral muscles** secondary to competitive antagonism of acetylcholine
- Can occur with OTC meds (even eye drops!) →Can be secondary to intentional overdose, inadvertent ingestion, medical noncompliance, or geriatric polypharmacy

Clinical Manifestations:

- **Flushing, dry skin, dry mucous membranes, mydriasis, fever, sinus tachycardia, functional ileus, urinary retention**, HTN, tremors, myoclonic, delirium, seizures, coma,
  - Hot as a hare – fever
  - Red as a beet – flushed skin
  - Blind as a bat – mydriasis
  - Dry as a bone – dry mouth and mucous membranes
  - Mad as a hatter – delirium
  - Full as a flask – urinary retention

Diagnosis:

- Mild toxicity – tachycardia, flushed face, dry mouth
- Moderate toxicity - Agitated delirium, hypertension, hyperthermia, urinary retention
- Severe toxicity - CNS depression, coma, seizures, arrhythmias (wide QRS and increased QT), rhabdomyolysis, hypotension
- Work up - **no test exists to check for anticholinergic levels**
  - Acetaminophen and salicylate screening - Order in all intentional poisonings
  - Blood and urine cultures – order in febrile patients
  - Serum chemistries, electrolyte analysis, ABG to assess for any acid-base disturbances
  - CT/MRI of head – especially if altered mental status, seizure, or coma
  - ECG – to assess for any cardiac arrhythmias

Treatment:

- Stop any causative agents
- Seizures – benzos used

- Hyperthermia – cooling protocol as antipyretics are not successful
- If <1 hour, use single dose activated charcoal may be administered to minimize absorption
- AMS – control airway with endotracheal intubation with cuffed tube
- Antidote – **physostigmine salicylate**, a cholinesterase inhibitor, shown to reduce delirium
    - CI in pts with cardiac conduction disturbances

Acetaminophen Overdose

Summary: Ingestion of ≥7.5g of APAP in adults that may result in liver failure
S/S: Anorexia, N/V, RUQ pain
Dx: Serum APAP levels
Tx: N-Acetylcysteine

Pathophysiology:

- The toxic metabolite, N-acetyl-p-benzoquinone imine (NAPQI), is produced by the **cytochrome P-450 enzyme system in the liver**
- Increased risk – alcoholic liver disease and undernutrition due to increased levels of toxins
- Found in many OTC products as well as prescriptions

Clinical Manifestations:

- Anorexia, vomiting, nausea, **RUQ pain**
- Can progress to renal failure, **hepatotoxicity,** and/or pancreatitis

Diagnosis:

- Serum Acetaminophen levels – **acute oral dose ≥150 mg/kg** (~7.5g in adults) in a 24-hour period
- Use the Rumack-Matthew nomogram to estimate likelihood of hepatotoxicity
    - Looks at the time of ingestion and serum levels

Treatment:

- **Poor prognosis** if - pH <7.3 after treatment, INR >3, Sr Cr >2.6, hepatic encephalopathy, hypoglycemia, and/or thrombocytopenia
- Antidote - **N-Acetylcysteine (NAC):** Glutathione precursor that increases hepatic glutathione stores to decreases levels of Acetaminophen
- Activated charcoal may also be used and some patients may require liver transplantation

Salicylate Poisoning

Summary: Salicylates impair cellular respiration by uncoupling oxidative phosphorylation
S/S: Acute vomiting, tinnitus, confusion, multiple organ failure (esp. renal)
Dx: Serum Salicylate levels >150 mg/kg; Metabolic acidosis and/or resp alkalosis
Tx: Activated charcoal +/- alkaline diuresis or hemodialysis

Pathophysiology:

- Salicylate tablets may form bezoars (tightly packed collection of partially diges8ted material in the stomach) which prolong absorption and toxicity - Symptoms can take days to develop
- Most concentrated salicylate - **Wintergreen** (methyl salicylate) – ANY exposure is serious
- Salicylates **impair cellular respiration** by uncoupling oxidative phosphorylation - Cause respiratory alkalosis and primary metabolic acidosis as the metabolites damage the mitochondria once in the cell

Clinical Manifestations:

- Acute overdose – vomiting, tinnitus, confusion, multiple organ failure (especially renal)
- Chronic overdose – nonspecific signs of confusion, AMS, hypoxia lactic acidosis, fever, hypotension

Diagnosis:

- Labs may show respiratory alkalosis, metabolic acidosis, high CK (in rhabdomyolysis)
- **Serum Salicylate levels >150 mg/kg** indicate severe toxicity (therapeutic range is 10-20 mg/dL)

Treatment:

- **Activated charcoal** is given ASAP
- Alkaline diuresis or **hemodialysis** → helps to eliminate salicylate
- Sodium Bicarbonate is often given for metabolic acidosis

Organophosphate Poisoning

Summary: Common insecticides that if ingested, can irreversibly bind to cholinesterase
S/S: Muscarinic and nicotinic manifestations
Dx: Atropine trial Symptoms improve with 1mg Atropine
Tx: Atropine for respiratory issues; pralidoxime for neuromuscular toxicity

Pathophysiology:

- **Commonly from insecticides**
  - MC associated with poisoning – chlorpyrifos, diazinon, dursban, fenthion, malathion, parathion
- Inhibit cholinesterase activity, causing acute muscarinic infections and some nicotinic symptoms
- Absorbed in GI tract, lungs, and skin and inhibit plasma and RBC cholinesterase to prevent the breakdown of acetylcholine. They can **irreversibly bind to cholinesterase**
- Can be used to reverse neuromuscular blockade and treat both Myasthenia Gravis and Alzheimer's Disease -Neostigmine, Pyridostigmine, Edrophonium

Clinical Manifestations:

- **Muscarinic** – diarrhea, lacrimation, salivation, emesis, bradycardia, bronchospasm, miosis, urination
- Nicotinic – muscle fasciculations, neuropathy, weakness

Diagnosis:

- Clinical
- **Atropine trial - Give 1mg and see if muscarinic symptoms improve or dissipate**
- Measure RBC acetylcholinesterase level indicates some level of poisoning

Treatment:

- Respiratory issues (bronchospasm/bronchorrhea) – **atropine**
- Neuromuscular toxicity – **IV Pralidoxime** (2-PAM) (given after atropine)
  - A nerve gas antidote that can bind to acetylcholinesterase to reactivate the enzyme
- Supportive therapy and decontamination also necessary

Ethylene Glycol Poisoning

Summary: Ingestion of automotive antifreeze leads to CNS depressive effects
S/S: Can be life threatening and cause renal failure, respiratory distress, seizures, coma
Dx: Clinical Dx; Urine may have calcium oxalate crystals
Tx: Supportive care to correct acidosis plus ethanol or fomepizole

Pathophysiology:

- Found in automotive **antifreeze** and can be ingested – absorbed via stomach and small intestine
- Has CNS depressive effects – oxidative reactions convert ethylene glycol to glycolaldehyde and glycolic acid – lactate is produced, causing metabolic acidosis –glyoxylic acid is converted into oxalic acid and glycine – oxalic acid is deposited as **calcium oxalate crystals** in tissues

Clinical Manifestations:

- **Symptoms of inebriation without alcohol**, nausea, vomiting
- More serious symptoms – carpopedal spasm, oliguria/anuria, ARF, respiratory distress, seizures, coma

Diagnosis:

- **Clinical diagnosis** – no correlation between serum ethylene glycol levels and severity of poisoning
- Calculate anion and osmolar gaps
- Urine – **calcium oxalate crystals**, RBC, myoglobin casts

Treatment:

- Supportive care – **correct acidemia** w/sodium bicarbonate; may require hemodialysis
- **Ethanol or fomepizole**

ADHD, AUTISM & OTHER DEVELOPMENTAL DISORDERS

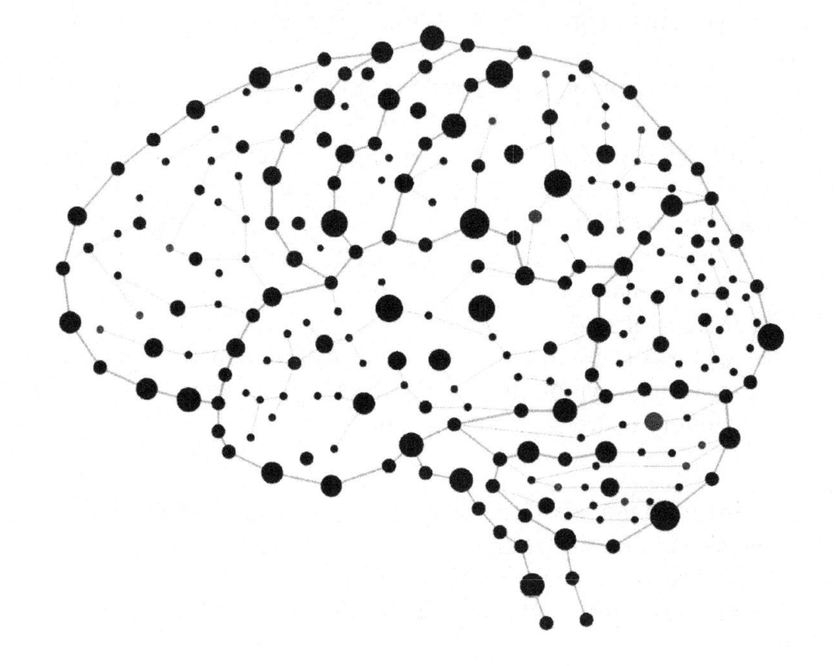

Attention Deficit Hyperactivity Disorder

Summary: Neurodevelopmental disorder associated w/ hyperactivity & inattention
S/S: Inability to concentrate or finish tasks, impatience, fidgeting, etc.
Dx: Must have ≥6 symptoms (≥5 symptoms if ≥17 years old) present for > 6 mo before 12 yo
Tx: Stimulants (methylphenidate, amphetamine) 1st line; atomoxetine

Pathophysiology:

- Attention & interpretation begins in the reticular system in the brainstem. The prefrontal cortex receives inputs from the brainstem arousal systems, and its function is particularly dependent on its neurochemical environment. The neurotransmitters **dopamine and NE** are linked to ADHD
- A neurodevelopmental disorder with onset in childhood (usually before age 12) and causes impairment in day-to-day life
- Attention – cognitive process through which the brain identifies stimuli within the context of time and space and selects what is relevant for both input and output
- Risk factors – M>F, family history, **low birth weight**, head trauma, OSA, lead exposure, iron deficiency, **prenatal exposure to alcohol/tobacco/cocaine**

Clinical Manifestations:

- 3 categories – inattentive, hyperactive/impulsive, and combined (mixed)
    - **Inattentive:** Wandering off task, lacking persistence, having difficulty focusing, and being disorganized and is NOT due to defiance or lack of comprehension
    - **Hyperactive/Impulsive**: Excessive motor activity when it is not appropriate. **Impulsivity** refers to making rushed decisions without forethought
- Adults will present with inability to concentrate/complete tasks, mood swings, impatience, inability to maintain relationships, restlessness, fidgetiness
- In school, children are unable to finish assignments, often missing their materials, seem impatient, frequently speak out of turn during class and answer questions before the question is completely stated. They often annoy their classmates by not waiting their turn in line or while playing games, violating rules, etc.
    - Children with inattentive symptoms, are often undiagnosed whereas the hyperactive children draw attention due to their behavior
    - Over 50% of children have a good prognosis. Poorer prognostic indicators include coexisting low intelligence,

aggressiveness, social/interpersonal problems, substance abuse, history of arrest, suicide attempts, etc.

Diagnosis:

- DSM-5 – ≥6 symptoms (≥5 symptoms if ≥17 yrs old) present for at least ≥6 mo before age 12:
- **Vanderbilt Assessment Scale - ADHD specific rating scale**
- Qb testing – not required but helpful for diagnosis

Inattentiveness	Hyperactivity/Impulsivity
Easily distracted	Fidgets with hands or squirms feet
Does not pay attention to details and makes careless mistakes	Leaves seat often and cannot sit still
Forgetful in daily activities	Runs about or climbs excessively
Does not listen when spoken to directly	Difficulty playing quietly
Does not follow instructions or finish tasks	Always on the go
Has difficulty organizing tasks/activities	Talks excessively
Avoids, dislikes, or refuses to engage in tasks that require sustained mental effort for a long period of time	Blurts out answers, often before questions are completed
Loses things necessary for tasks/activities	Difficulty waiting their turn
Sustaining attention is extremely difficult	Interrupts/intrudes on others

- Imaging:
  - MRI shows prefrontal cortex, basal ganglia, and cerebellum either are reduced in size or have abnormalities in asymmetry
  - Functional MRI shows hypoperfusion in prefrontal & basal ganglia regions

Treatment:

- **Psychotherapy** is effective, especially when used in conjunction with medications
- 1st line – **Stimulant drugs** (methylphenidate or amphetamines)
- Non-stimulant drugs (atomoxetine, bupropion, clonidine, guanfacine, viloxazine)

Editor's note – Untreated ADHD can significantly impede academic success and have social/work implications. These are also highly controlled and addictive substance. Consider getting formal testing (typically Qb testing) and UDS prior to initiation. It is important that we recognize both the risk of stimulant medications and the risk of not treating ADHD appropriately during formative years.

Autism Spectrum Disorder

Summary: Neurodevelopmental disorder associated with low social interaction, repetitive behavior, uneven intellect
S/S: Avoids eye contact, prefers to be alone, upset with minor routine changes, etc.
Dx: Must have > 2 sx associated with autism; MCHAT questionnaire utilized
Tx: Behavioral/language therapy

Pathophysiology:

- Theories include altered neuronal/axonal structure, neuron network disorganization in prefrontal/temporal cortices, large amount of small diameter axons in prefrontal cortex, neuron sizes (smaller in limbic system and larger in amygdala)
  - Alterations in face processing system (mediates eye gaze and facial cues) and mirror neuron network (mediates higher social cognition like interpreting intention of others)
- Risk factors – M >F, **rubella infection in pregnancy**, hypoxia (birth complications), advanced maternal or paternal age at time of conception, family history
  - *NOT* vaccinations (strong evidence)
- Autism Spectrum – 1/3 have verbal difficulties, 1/3 have intellectual disabilities
  - "Asperger's" - language and cognitive development less affected
    - The DSM-5 removed Asperger's disorder as its own distinct classification and replaced it with a general diagnosis of scalable severity of autism spectrum disorder. The term "Asperger's" may at times be used by those diagnosed prior to the adoption of the DSM-5.
  - Pervasive Developmental Disorder- Not Otherwise Specified (PDD-NOS) - Atypical autism or mild autism where the child does not fully meet criteria for "classic" autism

Clinical Manifestations:

- Neurodevelopmental disorder – **impaired social interaction, repetitive and stereotypic behavior, and uneven intellectual development**
- Patients often have difficulty processing social cues/body gestures, generating facial expressions, underdeveloped communication skills, affected speech
- Other characteristics – patients **avoid eye contact, prefer to be alone**, echolalia (repeat what they hear), have limited interests, are nonverbal or have delayed language, are **upset with minor routine changes (prefer familiarity),** unusual/intense reactions to light, colors, textures, tastes, sounds, and have fixated interests

- Symptoms may develop as early as at 2-3 years old

Diagnosis:

- Suspect in patients who have difficulty with reciprocating social-emotion, nonverbal communication, and developing, maintaining, and understanding relationships
- DSM-5 – symptoms must be present in the early developmental period and not be better explained by an intellectual developmental disorder/disability
    - **Persistent deficits in social interaction/communication**:
        - Deficits in social interaction reciprocity/failure to initiate/respond
        - Deficits in nonverbal communication behaviors used for social interaction (ex. abnormal eye contact/facial expression)
        - Deficits in forming/maintaining/understanding relationships; absence of interest in their peers
    - **Restricted & repetitive behaviors, interests, and/or activities**:
        - Stereotyped or repetitive motor movements, speech, or use of objects
        - Insistence on sameness, routine, ritualized patterns, or verbal nonverbal behavior
        - Highly restricted/fixated interests in abnormal intensity or focus
        - Either hyperreactive or hyporeactive to sensory stimulus
- **M-CHAT** (Modified Checklist for Autism in Toddlers) – 20 question checklists
    - Low risk 0-2 (<24 months, screen again at 2 years old)
    - Medium risk 3-7 (follow up)
    - High risk 8-20 (refer ASAP)

Treatment:

- 1st line – **Behavioral/language therapy** for an average of 30-40 hours/week
    - Picture exchange communication system to help build vocab to articulate observations, feelings, and desires, through pictures
    - Tips - let patients use pen/pencil/tablet to touch letters/pictures and the tablet speaks for them
- Requires substantial support from loved ones
- Pharmacologic treatment – can help with symptoms
    - Atypical antipsychotics (risperidone, aripiprazole) may help to reveal behavior problems (rituals, aggressiveness)
    - SSRIs can help with self-injury, mood, and outburst behaviors.
    - Stimulants for impulsivity and inattention

Conduct Disorder

Summary: Children <18 yo who act out, causing harm, w/o any guilt or remorse
S/S: Bullying, physical cruelty, property destruction, animal cruelty, aggression
Dx: <18 years old and ≥3 of the DSM 5 criteria in last 12 months plus ≥1 in the last 6 months
Tx: Psychotherapy for behavior mod; many meds are used to help manage sx

Pathophysiology:
- Etiology – Mix of genetic and environmental factors (parent w/ substance abuse issues)
  - Can still occur in high-functioning and healthy families
- Risk factors – Children (age <18) **with social/academic difficulties, lack of remorse**, defies authority, **M>F**
- Considered a **precursor to antisocial personality disorder** in adulthood - Over 40% of patients
- High comorbidity rate – ADHD, learning disability, mood disorders, substance use disorders

Clinical Manifestations:
- **Patients violate the rights of others and defy age-appropriate societal norms/rules**
- Lack empathy towards how their actions may affect others
- Aggression is common – Bullying, making threats, physical cruelty/animal cruelty, forcing sexual activity; destruction of property, lying, stealing, arson, physical aggression, running away from home
- Suicidal ideation is common in this patient population

Diagnosis:
- DSM-5 – **<18** in age & has done **≥3** of the following in the last **12 months** plus **≥1** in last **6 months:**
  - Aggression toward people and animals
  - Destroy property
  - Deceitfulness, lying, stealing
  - Serious violations of parental rules

Treatment:
- Environmental/**behavioral modifications with psychotherapy**; family therapy also helpful
- **Medications used to help improve symptoms** of impulsivity and unstable mood
  - Stimulants, bupropion, clonidine, lithium, antipsychotics, valproic acid for aggression
  - SSRIs may aid impulsivity and mood lability/irritability

Oppositional Defiant Disorder

Summary: Children <18 years old who argue, are defiant, and angry w/o causing severe harm
S/S: Persistent pattern of negative and hostile behavior towards adults
Dx: Children with ≥4 of the above symptoms for at least 6 months w/o severe aggression
Tx: Reward based behavior modification taught in psychotherapy

Pathophysiology:

- Symptoms begin at around age 8 but **may progress to conduct disorder in adulthood**
- High comorbidity with substance abuse disorders, mood disorders, ADHD
- Most prevalent in children from **families who have a lot of conflict** (loud, violent arguments)

Clinical Manifestations:

- **Persistent pattern of negative, hostile, and defiant behavior** towards adults - Irritability
- Symptoms – lack of social skills, lose temper easily, argue with and defy adults, break rules, annoy others deliberately, blame others for their mistakes, are easily annoyed, are spiteful/vindictive

Diagnosis:

- DSM-5 – Children with **≥4** of the above symptoms for at **least 6 months WITHOUT severe aggression**

Treatment:

- Family intervention and psychotherapy (**Reward based behavior modification**) – 1st line
- Treat any underlying depression or anxiety with SSRIs

PERSONALITY DISORDERS

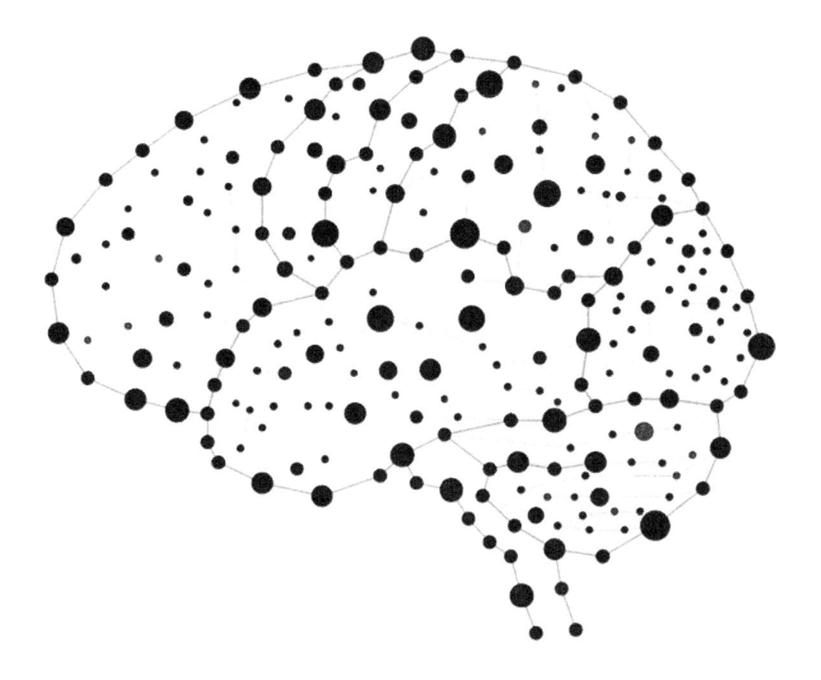

Personality traits – Stable patterns of thinking, perceiving, reacting, and relating

- Personality disorders – Traits become rigid and excessive, so much that social/occupational functioning is impaired. Usually develop in early adulthood
    - Cluster A – Odd/eccentric – Schizoid, Schizotypal, Paranoid
    - Cluster B – Dramatic/erratic – Antisocial, Borderline, Histrionic, Narcissistic
    - Cluster C – Anxious/fearful – Avoidant, Dependent, Obsessive-compulsive
    - Schizoid Personality Disorder (Cluster A)

> 3 W's (memory aid)
> Cluster A - weird
> Cluster B - wild
> Cluster C - worried

Schizoid Personality Disorder (Cluster A)

Summary: Isolation, restricted emotions 2ndary to neglect or trauma
S/S: Detached, distant, unbothered, dull, lack of desire to form relationships
Dx: Must have 4 of the symptoms to be diagnosed
Tx: Psychotherapy, mainly social skills training

Pathophysiology:

- Unknown cause, thought that genetics/environment play a role; may be caused by h/o **trauma or perinatal injury**
- Risk factors – Individuals **neglected as a child**, M>F, schizophrenia, major depression, anxiety, often have other personality disorders (schizotypal, paranoid, borderline, avoidant)

Clinical Manifestations:

- Limited range of emotional expression, pervasive pattern of **detachment, anhedonia, cold flat affect, isolated, and lifelong voluntary social withdrawal**
- Isolated
- Detached, distant (lack desire to be close to people and possesses little to no social skills)
- Unbothered by what others think of them – indifferent to praise/criticism
- Dull, humorless, rarely show emotion
- Less enjoyment out of bodily experiences; decreased libido
- React inappropriately to life events and appear as if they have no direction in their life

Diagnosis:

- DSM-5 – Pervasive pattern of detachment from social relationships and a restricted range of expression of emotions in interpersonal settings, beginning by early adulthood and present in a variety of contexts, as indicated by **4+ of the following**:
    - Neither desires nor enjoys close relationships, including being part of a family
    - Almost always chooses solitary activities
    - Has little, if any pleasure in sexual experiences with another person
    - Takes pleasure in few, if any, activities
    - Lacks close friends or confidants other than 1st degree relatives
    - Appears indifferent to the praise and criticism of others
    - Shows emotional coldness, detachment, or flattened affectivity

Treatment:

- Psychotherapy is 1st line

        - **Social skills training** through group therapy
    - Not very responsive to drugs Medications can be used to target anxiety/ depression – SSRIs

Schizotypal Personality Disorder (Cluster A)

Summary: Childhood disorder w/ odd thinking, disorganization, and paranoia
S/S: Cognitive and perceptual problems, interpersonal problems, and oddness
Dx: Must have 5 of the symptoms to be diagnosed
Tx: Psychotherapy is 1st line; medication can be used short term in low doses (antipsychotics)

Pathophysiology:

- Etiology – Thought to be environmental, learned behaviors, changes in brain, genetics
  - Environment may play a role, dysregulation of dopaminergic pathway; catechol-O-methyltransferase, which is involved in the degradation of synaptic dopamine; linked to schizophrenia
- Risk factors – Family history, **personal history of schizophrenia or another psychotic disorder**, M>F
- Begins in **childhood** and is typically chronic

Clinical Manifestations:

- Characterized by **cognitive and perceptual problems (paranoia or "magical thinking"), interpersonal problems (anxiety), disorganization & oddness**
  - Odd thinking and speech
  - Eccentric
  - Magical thinking (superstitious, telepathy, sixth sense, bizarre fantasies)
  - Ideas of reference: these individuals may think events relate to them in an important way and they may believe they have control over other people who are doing ordinary things
  - Unusual perceptions: may think others are out to get them
  - Anxiety
  - Have trouble relating to people (feel like they don't belong); minimal close friends (typically just family)
  - Often unkempt dress; odd/atypical mannerisms
  - Lack of understanding of social cues; may act inappropriately

Diagnosis:

- A pervasive pattern of social & interpersonal deficits marked by acute discomfort with, & reduced capacity for, close relationships as well as by cognitive or perceptual distortions & eccentricities of behavior, beginning by early adulthood, as indicated by **5+ of the following**:

- Odd beliefs or magical thinking influencing behavior and is inconsistent with subcultural norms (superstition, belief of clairvoyance, telepathy, "6th sense")
- Children and adolescents - bizarre fantasies or preoccupations
- Unusual perceptual experiences, including bodily illusions
- Odd thinking and speech
- Suspicious or paranoid ideation
- Inappropriate or constricted affect
- Behavior or appearance that is odd, eccentric, or peculiar
- Lack of close friends or confidants other than 1st degree relatives
- Social anxiety that does not diminish with familiarity and tend to have paranoid fears

Treatment:

- **Psychotherapy** is 1st line – Build a supportive relationship
  - CBT focuses on acquiring social skills & managing anxiety
- Short term & low dose atypical (2nd generation) antipsychotic drugs
- Antidepressants

Paranoid Personality Disorder (Cluster A)

Summary: A disorder w/ paranoia, mistrust, and suspicion of motives of others
S/S: Suspicious person who distrusts others and can be very violent
Dx: Must have 4 or more of the paranoia symptoms that begin in early adulthood
Tx: CBT; no proven treatment

Pathophysiology:

- Combination of biological, genetic, social, psychological causes but unknown
- Risk factors – M>F, increased among **1st degree biological relatives with schizophrenia and delusional disorder** (persecutory type), abuse during childhood

Clinical Manifestations:

- **Disorder of paranoia, mistrust, & suspiciousness of others' motives**
- Very suspicious, looks for hidden meanings in gestures & conversations
- Distrust others and feel they have been treated unfairly or lied to
- Described as cold, jealous, secretive, and serious
- Resentful and bear grudges
- Place a high premium on autonomy and react in a hostile manner if someone controls them
- Can have a bad temper, be irritable, and violent
- Hypervigilant
- Preoccupied with the belief that friends, family, and romantic partners are untrustworthy and unfaithful
- Detached and socially isolated

Diagnosis:

- DSM-5 – Pervasive distrust/suspiciousness that begins in early adulthood with **≥4 symptoms:**
  - Suspects others are trying to harm, deceive, or exploit them
  - Preoccupied with unjustified doubts of unloyalty/distrust
  - Won't confide in others
  - Reads hidden demeaning in benign remarks
  - Bears grudges
  - Perceives attack on their character/reputation
  - Recurrent suspicions without justification regarding fidelity of their spouse

- Treatment:
  - **CBT** – Individual/group therapy is the treatment of choice
  - Treat symptoms as there is no proven treatment for paranoid personality disorder

- Atypical/second-generation antipsychotics may decrease paranoia and severe agitation
- Antidepressants

Antisocial Personality Disorder (Cluster B)

Summary: Characterized by blatant disregard for consequences and lack empathy
S/S: Justify reckless behavior w/o remorse, destructive tendencies, unlawful acts
Dx: Must have at least 3 symptoms that began at age 15; Diagnosed at age 18
Tx: Psychotherapy is mainstay of treatment; meds include lithium, valproate, SSRIs

Pathophysiology:

- Widely unknown; developmental problems, brain differences (reduced activity in prefrontal cortex), genetics, and/or environmental factors all play a role
  - Strongest theory is that there is an abnormal serotonin transporter function
- Risk factors – M>F, those with **substance use disorder**, increased risk in first degree relatives, poor urban areas, prisoners, bullying, **conduct disorder as a child** (strongest RF)
- Patients may also have impulse control disorder, ADHD, and/or borderline personality disorder

Clinical Manifestations:

- **Pervasive pattern of disregard for consequences and for the rights of others**
  - Justify/rationalize their behavior, blame the victim for being foolish or helpless, and are indifferent to how their actions affect others
- Tend to have destructive tendencies, a manipulative nature and incessantly lie
- **Lack of remorse and empathy**
- Power-seeking behavior
- Repeatedly performs unlawful acts (destroy property, harass others, steal, etc.)
- Reckless disregard for safety of self or others (speed when driving, DWI)
- Impulsivity and failure to plan ahead – may suddenly change jobs, homes
- Arrogant self-appraisal
- Irritability and aggression – repeated physical fights or assaults
- Rationalize their actions by blaming those they hurt (i.e. "they deserved it") or the way life is ("unfair")
- Inability to maintain close personal relationships
- Negative job performance
- Socially and financially irresponsible

Diagnosis:

- DSM-5 – A pervasive pattern of disregard for and violation of the rights of others, **occurring since age 15**, as indicated **by 3+ of the following** in someone who is **AT LEAST 18 years old**:
    - Failure to conform to social norms with respect to lawful behaviors, as indicated by repeatedly performing acts that are grounds for arrest
    - Deceitfulness, as indicated by repeated lying, manipulation, use of aliases, or conning others for personal profit or pleasure
    - Impulsivity or failure to plan ahead
    - Irritability & aggressiveness as indicated by repeated physical fights or assaults
    - Reckless disregard for safety of self or others
    - Consistent irresponsibility (not paying bills)
    - Not feeling remorse, as indicated by being indifferent to or rationalizing having hurt, mistreated, or stolen from another

Treatment:

- **CBT** – Addiction and family counseling also used to treat co-existing disorders
    - Contingency management - Positive reinforcement with good behavior
- Aggressive patients with prominent impulsivity and labile affect – **lithium, valproate, SSRIs**
- Atypical antipsychotics (ex. risperidone or quetiapine) can help, but they are not commonly used
- Benzodiazepines are not recommended as they increase the risk of abuse & addiction

Borderline Personality Disorder (Cluster B)

Summary: Unstable relationships w/ fear of abandonment resulting in impulsivity
S/S: Patients do anything to avoid abandonment, even threaten suicide
Dx: Must have 5 or more symptoms that began in early adulthood
Tx: Dialectic behavioral therapy is 1st line

Pathophysiology:

- Multifactorial; strong theories include:
  - Genetically predisposed to enhanced anxiety, emotional liability, instability
  - Psychosocial (sexual, physical, and/or emotional abuse/neglect)
  - Neurobiological (serotonin dysfunction, reductions in the hippocampus and amygdala, disrupted frontal lobe functioning)
- Risk factors – F>M, coexisting disorder (depression, anxiety, PTSD, eating disorders, substance use), **sexual or physical abuse**, neglect as a child, **separation from caregivers, loss of a parent**
- High risk of attempting/completing suicide
- Frequently comorbid with PTSD

Clinical Manifestations:

- Pervasive pattern of **unstable personal relationships**, self-images, and emotions; often extremely impulsive, acting out in a sexual manner, excessive spending, parasuicidal gestures, and substance abuse
- "Borderline" = on the border between neurosis and psychosis
- Intolerance of being alone so they do anything to avoid abandonment and generate crisis
- Feelings of intense feel and anger if they feel they are being abandoned or neglected
- Idealize potential caregiver/lover early in the relationship and demand spending time together
- Impulsivity leading to self-harm (**suicidal behaviors and/or self-mutilation**)
- Patients often use "splitting" as a defense mechanism

- Diagnosis:
  - DSM-5 – A pervasive pattern of instability of interpersonal relationships, self-image, and emotions that is marked by impulsivity, beginning by early adulthood, as **indicated by 5 (or more) of the following**:
    - Frantic efforts to avoid real or imagined abandonment
    - Intense, unstable interpersonal relationships

        - Unstable self-image or sense of self
        - Impulsivity in at least 2 areas that are potentially harmful (sexual activity, substance use, binge eating, spending, etc.)
        - Recurrent suicidal threats or attempts at self-mutilation
        - Affective instability due to a marked reactivity of mood
        - Feelings of emptiness
        - Difficulty controlling anger
        - Transient, stress-related paranoid ideation or dissociative symptoms
    - McLean Screening Instrument and BSL-23 are sometimes used to help aid in diagnosis

- Treatment:
    - 1st line – **Dialectical Behavior Therapy (DBT)** which combines mindfulness practices with concrete interpersonal and emotion regulation skills
    - Systems Training for Emotional Predictability and Problem Solving (STEPPS) is also used - group sessions for 20 weeks where one is taught to manage emotions and care for themselves
    - Transference-focused psychotherapy, schema-focused therapy, and mentalization are all used
        - These are more focused forms of therapy for borderline personality disorder
    - Mood stabilizers – lamotrigine commonly used and can be helpful; valproic acid and carbamazepine: decrease irritability and aggressiveness; lithium carbonate: decreases anger, irritability, and self-mutilation
    - Antidepressants: SSRIs for mood fluctuations, aggression
    - Second generation antipsychotics reduce paranoid/psychotic ideation, impulsive aggression, and depression
    - BPD may not respond to medications, but can still treat the comorbidities. Patients frequently have a long history of many psychiatric medication trials/failures.

Histrionic Personality Disorder (Cluster B)

Summary: Patients w/ excessive emotion who are highly attention seeking
S/S: Use their physical appearance for attention; Often act out (sexual/provocative)
Dx: ≥ symptoms that begin in adulthood relating to excessive emotion and attention seeking
Tx: Psychodynamic psychotherapy; No efficacious treatment exists

Pathophysiology:

- Unknown etiology/pathophysiology
- Risk factors – F>M, comorbidities (antisocial, borderline, or narcissistic personality disorders), presence of somatic symptom disorder, MDD

Clinical Manifestations:

- Pervasive pattern of excessive emotion and attention seeking, "dramatic"
- **Use their physical appearance to gain the attention of others** (seductive or provocative)
- Tend to present themselves in a manner that will attract attention - **dressing in flashy/ revealing clothes, behave in ways that are flirtatious & seductive**
- May have difficulty achieving emotional intimacy in romantic or sexual relationships
- Without being aware of it, they often act out of a role (i.e. victim/ princess) in their relationships
- May seek to control partner through emotional manipulation or seductiveness on one level yet displaying a marked dependency on them at another level
- **Change friends and jobs frequently**

Diagnosis:

- DSM-5 – Pervasive pattern of excessive emotionality and attention seeking, beginning by early adulthood, as indicated by **5+ of the following:**
    - Uncomfortable in situations in which he or she is not the center of attention
    - Interaction with others is characterized by inappropriate sexually seductive/provocative behavior
    - Displays rapidly shifting/shallow expression of emotions
    - Consistently uses physical appearance to draw attention to self
    - Style of speech that is excessively impressionistic and lacking in detail

- Shows self-dramatization, theatricality, and exaggerated expression of emotion
- Is suggestible (i.e., easily influenced by others or circumstances)
- Considers relationships to be more intimate than they are

Treatment:

- Long-term psychotherapy with experienced therapist
    - **Psychodynamic psychotherapy** – focus on underlying conflicts
        - Supportive and logical approach to a patient's problems that requires sensitivity to their emotional concerns
- Medications may be used to manage symptoms of anger and/or impulsivity
- Little is known about efficacy of medications and/or CBT

Narcissistic Personality Disorder (Cluster B)

Summary: Characterized by grandiose characteristics, need for admiration, and lack of empathy
S/S: Consider themselves to be elite but have very fragile self-esteem
Dx: Must have 5 or more symptoms of narcissism that began during early adulthood
Tx: Intensive psychodynamic psychotherapy or CBT are common 1st line tx

Pathophysiology:

- Thought to be due to biological, genetic, social factors (i.e. how a person interacts in early development with their family, friends and other children)
- Psychological factors also play a role - Individual's personality and temperament, shaped by their environment and learned coping skills to deal with stress
- Risk factors – M>F, family history, **caregiver that was extremely critical or excessively praised, admired, and/or indulged the patient as a child**
- Comorbidities may include depressive disorder, eating disorder, substance use disorder (esp. cocaine), another personality disorder

Clinical Manifestations:

- Characterized by a **long-standing pattern of grandiosity** (either in fantasy or actual behavior), an overwhelming **need for admiration**, and typically a **complete lack of empathy** toward others
- Have difficulty regulating their self-esteem so they need praise and to be affiliated with special people or institutions (very fragile self-esteem so they watch to see what others think of them)
- Need to maintain a **sense of superiority**
- Believe they are of primary importance in everybody's life (to anyone they meet)
- Snobbish, disdainful, condescending, or patronizing attitudes (i.e. may complain about a clumsy waiter's "rudeness" or "stupidity")
- Grandiose sense of importance, preoccupation with unlimited success, belief that one is special/unique, exploitive of others, lack of empathy, arrogance, and jealous of others
- Overestimation of their own worth and underestimation of the achievements/worth of others

Diagnosis:

- DSM-5 – A pervasive pattern of grandiosity (in fantasy or behavior), need for admiration, and lack of empathy, beginning by early adulthood, as indicated **by 5+ of the following**:

- Has a grandiose sense of self-importance, preoccupied with fantasies of unlimited success, power, brilliance, beauty, or ideal love
- Believes that he or she is "special" and unique and can only be understood by, or should associate with, other special or high-status people (or institutions)
- Requires excessive admiration
- Has a sense of entitlement
- Is interpersonally exploitative
- Lacks empathy – unwilling to recognize or identify with the feelings and needs of others
- Is often envious of others or believes that others are envious of him or her
- Shows arrogant, haughty behaviors or attitudes

Treatment:

- May not seek help; when these individuals seek help, it is likely for the anger or depression they feel when deprived of something they feel entitled to, such as a promotion – "Narcissistic injury"
- 1st line – **Intensive psychodynamic psychotherapy** to focus on underlying conflict
- Cognitive-behavioral psychotherapy may work because patients are able to "increase mastery" and they seek to have their therapist admire their behavior

Avoidant Personality Disorder (Cluster C)

Summary: Avoid interacting with others due to fear of rejection, criticism, humiliation
S/S: Need to be liked, isolation, low self-confidence, preoccupied w/ rejection
Dx: ≥ 4 or more symptoms of social inhibition, feeling inadequate, and hypersensitivity to criticism
Tx: Psychotherapy is 1st line; meds used to manage sx

Pathophysiology:

- Thought to be a combo of genetics, psychological, and environmental factors as are majority of the personality disorders
- Risk factors – harm avoidance, child abuse, parental neglect, trauma, uncaring caregiver, **anxiety as a child, experiences of rejection**
  - Men and women affected equally
- Comorbidities may include MDD, OCD, anxiety disorder, and/or another personality disorder (particularly dependent or borderline)
- Has been detected in children as early at 2 years old

Clinical Manifestations:

- Characterized by **avoidance of social situations or interactions that involve risk of rejection, criticism, or humiliation**
- Experience a need to be liked in order to build a relationship or go around people
  - Refuse a promotion in fear of criticism, avoid meetings, avoid making new friends
- Assume people will be critical and disapprove of them
- **Long for interaction** but avoid occupational, social, and academic functions secondary to fear of disapproval
- Blush easily, stutter, or remain silent during conversations
- Low self-confidence and very sensitive to rejection
- Feeling unwanted and undesirable
- Preoccupation with rejection
- Self-isolating behavior
- **Inferiority complex** – desire relationships but avoids them due to feelings of inadequacy, sensitivity to criticism, and fear of rejection and humiliation

Diagnosis:

- DSM-5 – A pervasive pattern of social inhibition, feelings of inadequacy, and hypersensitivity to negative evaluation, beginning in early adulthood, as indicated by **4+ of the following**:
  - Avoids occupational activities that involve significant interpersonal contact because of fears of criticism, disapproval, or rejection

- Is unwilling to get involved with people unless certain of being liked
- Shows restraint within intimate relationships because of the fear of being shamed or ridiculed
- Is preoccupied with being criticized or rejected in social situations
- Is inhibited in new interpersonal situations because of feelings of inadequacy
- Views self as socially inept, personally unappealing, or inferior to others
- Is unusually reluctant to take personal risks or to engage in any new activities because they may prove embarrassing

Treatment:

- Treatment is not normally sought until it begins to interfere with activities of daily living
- 1st line treatment: **Psychotherapy** – behavioral and group therapy to focus on social skills
- SSRIs to help with depressive/isolation symptoms, beta blockers for the performance anxiety component

Dependent Personality Disorder (Cluster C)

Summary: Characterized by fear of abandonment and inability to care for oneself
S/S: Clingy, submissive, reactive behavior toward caregiver, fear of independence
Dx: Must have 5 or more symptoms of submissive behavior and fear of separation
Tx: Individual psychotherapy

Pathophysiology:

- Genetics, biological factors and psychological (developmental or environmental) factors play a role
- Etiology – Thought to be due to a **childhood environment in which dependent behaviors were directly or indirectly rewarded**, independent activities were discouraged, and/or increasing evidence from twin studies also suggests possible genetic influence.
- Risk factors – cultural factors, negative experiences as a child, and familial presence of anxiety or a personality disorder increases risk
- Increased **traits of submissiveness, separation insecurity, and anxiousness**
- Comorbidities – MDD, anxiety, alcohol use disorder, other personality disorder (borderline, histrionic)

Clinical Manifestations:

- Predominantly submissive, reactive, and clinging behavior that is characterized by the **need to be taken care of due to fear of abandonment**
- Reacts with increasing appeasement and submissiveness and **urgently seeks a replacement relationship to provide caregiving and support**
- Truly do not feel like they can take care of themselves
- Consider themselves inferior and belittle their abilities
- Have a strong need for reassurance and approval and may appear childlike and clinging
- Characterized by feelings of inadequacy, hypersensitivity to criticism, and a need for reassurance
- Disorder has a pattern of seeking and maintaining connections to important others, rather than avoiding and withdrawing from relationships; interact socially only with the few they depend on

Diagnosis:

- DSM-5 – A pervasive and excessive need to be taken care of that leads to submissive and clinging behavior and fears of separation, beginning by early adulthood, as indicated by **5+ of the following:**

- Has difficulty making everyday decisions without excessive amount of reassurance from others
- Needs others to assume responsibility for most major areas of their life
- Difficult disagreeing w/ others due fear of loss of support/approval
- Has difficulty initiating projects or doing things on his or her own
- Goes to excessive lengths to obtain nurturance and support from others (do unpleasant tasks)
- Feels uncomfortable/helpless when alone due to fear of being unable to care for themselves
- Urgently seek another relationship when a close relationship ends
- Is unrealistically preoccupied with fears of being left to take care of themself

Treatment:

- **Individual psychotherapy** is the most employed and studied modality
  - Focuses on examining fears of independence
- Pharmacological treatment of cluster c personality disorders is limited but can be used for symptom management
  - SSRI or tricyclic antidepressant therapy - For fatigue, malaise, vague anxiety
  - Impulsivity and aggression may respond to serotonergic medications
  - Instability and lability may respond to serotonergic or dopaminergic medications
  - Psychotic-like experiences may respond to antipsychotics
- Avoid benzodiazepines due to increased risk of addiction

Obsessive Compulsive Personality Disorder (Cluster C)

Summary: Rigid perfectionism, perseveration, intimacy avoidance, restricted affect
S/S: Obsession w/ perfectionism interfering w/ ability to complete social and/or occupational tasks
Dx: ≥4 symptoms of preoccupation w/ orderliness, perfectionism, and inflexibility
Tx: Psychodynamic therapy; SSRIs may be helpful

Pathophysiology:

- Increase in **serotonin activity** has been associated with perfectionism and compulsivity
- Etiology – results from combination of, and interaction between, temperament (genetic and other biological factors) and psychological (developmental or environmental) factors
- **Compulsivity, oppositional behavior, restricted expression of emotion, and intimacy problems have all been shown to be moderately heritable**
- Comorbidities may include MDD and alcohol use disorder

Clinical Manifestations:

- Characterized by the **desire to be orderly perfect, and have complete control with no room for flexibility that prevents one from completing a task or being productive**; goal is perfection
    - *Differentiation from OCD*: OCPD does not include obsessions with compulsions
- 4 traits: rigid perfectionism (required), perseveration, intimacy avoidance, and restricted affectivity
- Symptoms may lessen with time but can last long term
- Empathy is somewhat impaired; lack interest in the ideas, feelings, or behavior of others
- Focus on rules, details, schedules, lists, etc. and repeatedly check for mistakes; plan ahead in great detail and dislike/will not make any changes; feel they have time to relax or see friends; do not work well in groups, make detailed lists about how things should be done, often behind schedule; intimacy may be impaired because relationships may be seen as secondary to work/productivity; comply with all rules set by the authorities with no exceptions
- Self-critical
- Patients often experience fatigue, malaise, and anxiety

Diagnosis:

- DSM-5 – A pervasive pattern of preoccupation with orderliness, perfectionism, and mental and interpersonal control, at the expense of flexibility, openness, and efficiency, beginning by early adulthood, as indicated by **4+ of the following:**
    - Preoccupied with details, rules, lists, order, organization, or schedules to the extent that the major point of the activity is lost
    - Shows perfectionism that interferes with task completion
    - Excessively devoted to work and productivity and excludes leisure activities and friendships
    - Is overconscientious, scrupulous, and inflexible about matters of morality, ethics, or values (not accounted for by cultural or religious identification)
    - Unable to discard worn-out/ worthless objects even when they have no sentimental value
    - Reluctant to delegate tasks or to work with others unless they do things exactly as they say
    - Miserly spending style where money is viewed as being saved for future catastrophes
    - Rigid and stubborn

Treatment:

- **Psychodynamic therapy** and CBT – diminish the patient's excessive need for control and perfection
- SSRIs commonly used
- No proven effective treatments

SOMATIC SYMPTOM & RELATED DISORDER

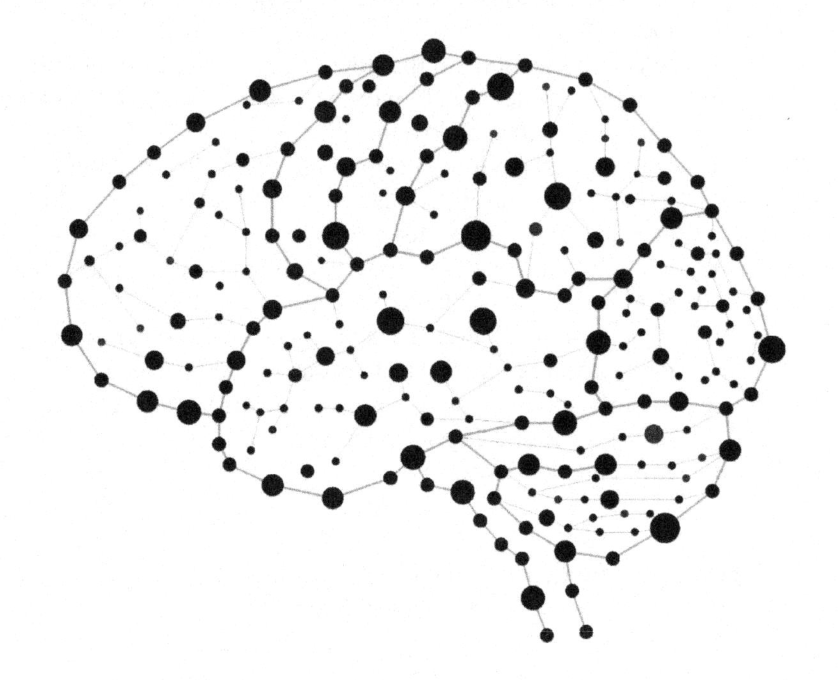

Factitious Disorder (Munchausen Syndrome)

Summary: Disorder in which one uses deception to falsify illness/injury on themselves or another
S/S: Patient will do anything to appear ill/impaired in suit of assuming a sick role
Dx: Falsification of sx or causing injury/disease w/deception, no secondary gain, for ≥6m
Tx: Psychotherapy – individual or family therapy; poor prognosis

Pathophysiology:

- Two main forms:
  - **Munchausen syndrome** – factitious disorder **imposed on self**
  - **Munchausen syndrome *by proxy*** – factitious disorder **imposed on another** (ex. mother on child)
- First presentation usually 3rd or 4th decade of life, although children have been diagnosed as well
- Risk factors – female sex, unmarried, **healthcare workers** (past and present)
- Pathogenesis not completely understood, but is associated with certain psychosocial factors, neurocognitive impairment, and neuroimaging abnormalities. Leading theories:
  - Search for nurturance - Induce illness in order to be cared for and nurtured. Often, they are caretakers themselves and use sickness as a means of role reversal so that they can be cared for
  - Secondary gains (Malingering) - Use of an illness to obtain disability benefits, to be excused from obligations such as work, and to gain the attention of family members
  - Need for power and superiority; feels clever and powerful after deceiving others
  - To obtain drugs – not necessarily for addiction, but rather the rush or thrill of fooling the health care provider
  - To create a sense of identity – poor sense of self but uses the sick role to establish an identity
  - To defend against anxiety or psychosis – severe anxiety over fears of abandonment or feeling powerless/helpless, sick role allows them to feel in control, powerful and cared for

Clinical Manifestations:

- Use **deceptive behaviors to consciously falsify physical or psychiatric symptoms or induce injury or disease upon themselves**. The patients intent is to appear ill, impaired, or injured
- Behavior is present in the absence of external rewards (i.e., insurance money) and is generally a means for the patient to fulfill a psychological need by assuming a sick role

- The patient can present complaining of essentially any general medical or psychiatric illness. Patients can be very **knowledgeable about medicine** and can go to extreme lengths to feign injury or illness
- MC falsified symptoms and diseases:
  - Abdominal pain, arthralgia, chest pain, coagulopathy, diarrhea, hematuria
  - Hypercortisolism, hyperthyroidism, hypoglycemia, infections, seizures
  - Skin wounds that won't heal, vomiting, weakness
  - Psychiatric - Bereavement, depression, psychosis, and suicidal ideation and/or behavior

- Methods patients use to feign illness:
  - **Exaggeration of symptoms/signs, psychological disturbances, illnesses**:
    - Administering medications (anticoagulants, insulin, laxatives, thyroid hormones), applying/ injecting contaminants (feces, bacteria, sputum), delaying wound healing (self-contamination, intentional dehiscence, or self- trauma), swallowing or instilling blood
  - **Fabricating medical history** or falsifying medical records
  - Aggravating genuine, existing illness by **not adhering to medical recommendations**
    - Not taking anticonvulsant meds to induce seizure, not taking insulin if diabetic
  - Presenting benign physical findings as pathological - Patient with a lifelong congenitally constricted pupil claiming it was caused by recent head trauma
  - Tampering with medical instruments, tests, or lab specimens

Diagnosis:
- DSM-5 – **Falsification of physical or psychological signs or symptoms, or induction of injury or disease, associated with identified deception for ≥6 months despite reassurance**
  - The individual presents himself or herself to others as ill, impaired, or injured
  - The deceptive behavior is evident even in the absence of obvious external rewards (malingering)
  - The behavior is not better explained by another disorder
- Can have a single episode or recurrent episodes
- Suspect factitious disorder in patients that have **high rates of healthcare utilization, are evasive or reluctant in providing medical history, refuse to grant access to prior medical record**, show inconsistency in the history, examination, and lab tests, have lengthy and extensive clinical evaluation that is negative, and

consistently show a poor response to standard treatments for the disease
- Imaging rarely done but neurocognitive findings include dysfunction in the right hemisphere of the brain (impairment with conceptual organization, management of complex information, and judgement)
    - MRI – disseminated white matter lesions bilaterally
    - CT – moderate bilateral frontotemporal cortical atrophy, mild cerebral atrophy, hyper perfusion of the right thalamus

Treatment:
- No specific pharmacologic treatments for factitious disorder, however underlying comorbidities should be treated appropriately
- **Individual Psychotherapy** – empathetic/supportive, should not be confrontational
- Family Therapy - Patients often come from dysfunctional families and act out because their needs aren't being met or they don't know how to properly express their needs
- SSRIs may be helpful
- Prognosis for factitious disorder imposed on self is generally poor especially if not caught early Prognosis of factitious disorder imposed on another is also poor. High mortality rate of victims
- Complications can include unnecessary surgical procedures and any related iatrogenic complications or accidental death from factitious behavior (inducing hypoglycemia, seizure, etc.)

Related diagnoses:
- **Malingering** – Similar to factitious disorder, malingering employs deceptive behavior to feign an illness, but the key difference is that there is an **obvious external benefit** that is the motivation for the behavior (ex. money, medication, time off work, or avoiding criminal prosecution)
    - Patients with factitious disorder are much more likely to undergo invasive or painful diagnostic or therapeutic procedures, while malingering patients will likely avoid them

- **Hypochondriasis** (also called **illness anxiety disorder**) – Excessive concern about either having or developing a serious undiagnosed disease
    - Patient experiences distress that primarily **comes from an unfounded fear of having some sort of disease, present for at least 6 months**, rather than having true alarming physical symptoms
    - Distress and fear persist despite normal physical exam findings and negative lab results
    - Most prevalent in young adults with both sexes affected equally
    - MC in those unemployed, without health insurance, and who are uneducated
    - Two subtypes of illness anxiety disorder:
        - **Care seeking type** are patients who frequent their doctor's office looking for additional testing

- **Care avoidance type** will tend to avoid all health care outlets unless necessary

Conversion Disorder

Summary: Neurological symptoms/deficits (motor or sensory) w/o neuro disease
S/S: Motor – paralysis, tremor, tics; Sensory – visual (MC), anesthesia, deafness
Dx: ≥1 symptom of altered motor/sensory function, not attributable to any Dx; NOT intentional
Tx: Education is the mainstay with therapeutic alliance with patients with PT/CBT

Pathophysiology:

- **MC in females** and onset is usually in adolescence or young adulthood
- Symptoms are a **consequence of emotional conflict**, with repression of conflict into the unconscious
- Risk factors - Rural populations, low socioeconomic status, lack of education, history of sexual or physical abuse, mental illness (depression, anxiety, schizophrenia, personality disorder)

Clinical Manifestations:

- **Neurological symptoms/deficits involving motor or sensory issues that develop unconsciously and are not linked to a neurological disease** – abnormal movement, weakness, nonepileptic seizures
  - Motor dysfx – paralysis, aphonia, mutism, seizures, gait, changes, involuntary movements, tics, weakness swallowing
  - Sensory dysfx –deafness, paresthesia, **visual changes** (MC)
- Onset is abrupt and exacerbation of sx often attributed to stress or trauma
- "Conversion" of psychic conflict into physical neurologic symptoms
- **Symptoms are NOT intentionally produced**

Diagnosis:

- DSM-5 – **≥1 symptom** of altered motor or sensory function, not attributable to any medical condition
  - Causes clinically significant distress or impairment in social/occupational function
- Nonepileptic vs. epileptic seizure – EEG and prolactin level are helpful (prolactin doubles in epilepsy)
  - Lack of postictal confusion, closed eyes during the seizure, ictal crying, and a fluctuating course can suggest nonepileptic seizures
- **Signs and symptoms are not usually consistent with the disease.** Patients may possess one symptom but not meet all criteria or symptoms vary. For example, a tremor may disappear if patient is distracted

Treatment:

- First-line treatment is **education** on the disorder, develop a **therapeutic alliance** – reassure patient sx are real despite definitive dx.
- Second-line treatment is **physical therapy** for motor sx and **CBT** for other sx including sensory sx.
- ¾ of patients have spontaneous resolution and ¼ may have recurrence
- Good prognostic factors – acute onset, short duration, high intelligence, identifiable stressor, male sex
- Treat any comorbid conditions

Somatic Symptom (Somatoform) Disorder

Summary: Psych disorder that manifests as a physical sx w/o medical reason
S/S: Excessive, dysfunctional thoughts about symptoms even with reassurance
Dx: Distressing symptoms that disrupt life ≥ 6 months that meet clinical criteria
Treatment: CBT is 1st line; reassurance/empathy; may use SSRI

Pathophysiology:

- Not known; possible psychosocial etiologies are typically the focus for most studies
    - Psychosocial etiology - **Cognitive behavioral model** is the most supported model. The disorder is characterized by increased and nonstop anxiety about threats to one's health
    - Some possible psychosocial etiologies for illness anxiety include incorrect assumptions about the prevalence and spread of certain diseases, overestimations of vulnerability, early family, and own childhood disease exposure (many more exist)
- Unexplained symptoms however remain a major component of conversion disorder and pseudocyesis (false belief of being pregnant)
- Usually begins before age 30
- **Common to comorbid psychiatric issues** (general anxiety disorder, dysthymia (persistent depressive), unipolar major depressive, phobias, and panic disorder). Also, **common to have a personality disorder** (obsessive compulsive, avoidant, and paranoid personality disorders MC)

Clinical Manifestations:

- Multiple physical complaints associated with **excessive, dysfunctional thoughts, feelings, and behaviors secondary to those symptoms**
- Any mental disorder that manifests as **physical symptoms that suggest illness or injury, but cannot be explained fully by a disorder or by the direct effect of a substance**
- Concern about acquiring an illness **despite normal physical exam, lab testing, and reassurance**
- Symptoms interfere with patients employment or relationships and are not under voluntary control
- Symptoms are persistent and patients worry about them enough that they consume their thoughts
- Some individuals having drastic effects on functioning. Some may assess their bodies multiple times a day by checking their pulse, blood pressure etc.

- **High healthcare utilization** – undergo excessive number of examination and lab testing. Patients may push their providers to prescribe more invasive testing. Often when a provider denies their requests for high risk and invasive procedures, they will "shop" around for a provider who will grant their wishes
- On the opposite end on the spectrum, some patients fear iatrogenic disorders and will try their best to avoid healthcare all together; they may look for diagnosis and alternative treatments online

Diagnosis:

- DSM-5 – Distressing symptoms that **disrupt life for ≥6 months** with one of the following:
    - Disproportionate and persistent thoughts about the symptoms and their seriousness
    - High anxiety about health/symptoms
    - Excessive time and energy spent on symptoms/health concerns
- Somatic symptoms are mild or nonexistent
- Illness preoccupation is not better explained by other mental disorders

Treatment:

- Any underlying general medical disorders must be addressed/ruled out and treated appropriately
- **CBT** has been shown to help by teaching stress management, distraction, and relaxation techniques
- Provide **reassurance**, empathize with patients, and address symptoms as real until proven otherwise
- **Fluoxetine and venlafaxine** have been shown to reduce symptoms
- Treat any comorbid psychiatric disorders

EATING DISORDERS & BODY-IMAGE RELATED DISORDERS

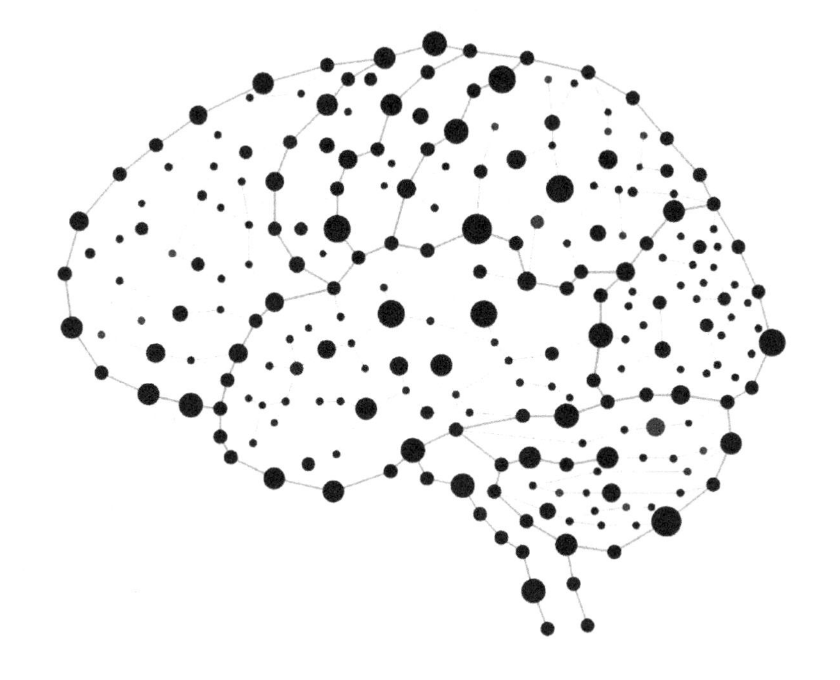

Anorexia Nervosa

Summary: Typically, thin teenage F fear of becoming obese due to societal norms
S/S: Severely restrict calories; Binge eat and then vomit/use laxatives in purging
Dx: Clinical dx, intentional restriction of food, refusal to maintain healthy BMI; exam may show lanugo, bradycardia, hypotension
Treatment: Unstable – hospitalization; Stable – CBT, SSRIs to help with mood and weight gain, may also include hospitalization

Pathophysiology:

- Malnutrition causes disruption of multiple organ systems
  - Estrogen mediated impairments in learning/memory cause cognitive inflexibility, weak central coherence/social emotional processing that can be from lack of energy - malnutrition causes cardiac muscle mass, chamber size, and output to decrease, therefor arrhythmias (prolonged QT) and murmurs (MVP) may occur
  - Amenorrhea can occur in thinner females due to adipose tissue contributes to estrogen so lack thereof can lead to hormonal imbalances causing amenorrhea
  - Endocrine abnormalities may occur – hypogonadism, hypothyroidism, increased cortisol

- Risk Factors – **Adolescents, F>M**, genetic, comorbid mood disorder (depression, OCD, social phobia), poor family dynamic, **middle/upper socioeconomic class**
  - Highest mortality rate of psychiatric disorders secondary only to opioid use disorder
  - *Editor's note – Eating disorders are frequently underdiagnosed in males; also frequently missed in overweight patients. Any BMI and demographic can have disordered eating. Be sure to not discount patients bc they are not the "most common" presentation.*

Clinical Manifestations:

- Patients are constantly **intentionally restriction food intake/trying to become thinner out of fear of weight gain, a distorted body image**
- Types
  - **Restrictive** – restrict food intake but do not binge/purge; some patients exercise excessively
  - **Binge eating/purging type** – episodes of binge eating or purging behavior (induce vomiting and/or misuse laxatives, enemas, diuretics)
- Symptoms to watch for –

        - **Dramatic weight loss**
        - Sleep problems
        - **Amenorrhea**
        - Preoccupied with weight/calories, patients may dress in layers, cook meals for others without eating, spend a lot of time studying diets and calories, avoid eating in public, burns calories taken in, intense fear of gaining weight even though they are thin

    - Physical exam
        - Hypotension
        - Bradycardia (can do a walking test to confirm its not from athletic conditioning as pts may claim)
        - HLD
        - **Lanugo** (fine hair all over body)

    - Labs: restrictive – may have no lab abnormalities until they are critically ill;
      binge-purge type – lab abnormalities are often present
        - Testing may reveal:
            - Hypokalemia and hyponatremia and hypercholesteremia – **metabolic alkalosis**
            - Prolonged QT intervals

Diagnosis:

- Clinical criteria
    - Restriction of energy intake relative to requirements leading to a significantly low body weight in the context of age, sex, developmental trajectory, and health
    - Intense fear of gaining weight or becoming fat
    - Disturbance in the way in which one's body weight or shape is experienced, undue influence of body weight or shape on self-evaluation
    - Denial of the seriousness of the current low body weight
- Severity
    - Mild: BMI ≥17
    - Mod: BMI 16-16.99
    - Severe: BMI 15-15.99
    - Extreme: BMI < 15
        - Anorexia nervosa and low BMI can be *fatal* due to nutritional imbalances, heart issues, etc.

Treatment:

- **Nutrition rehab and psychotherapy** – inpatient care if severe or unstable
    - Goal is to gain 1.5kg/week inpatient and 0.5kg/week outpatient

        - Always refer to therapy and registered dietician (with experience treating eating disorders when possible)
    - Psychiatric hospitalization, partial hospital and outpatient care
    - CBT and especially **family therapy** are very helpful
    - Can use SSRIs or atypical antipsychotics (**olanzapine** helps reduce anxiety and produce weight gain)
    - Caution – **refeeding syndrome** can occur if food is reintroduced too quickly
        - Have a low index of suspicion to refer to a higher level of care
        - Phosphate demand in starving body (severe hypophosphatemia)
        - Shifts in electrolytes can cause seizures, heart failure, coma, etc. Carefully monitor electrolytes and slowly increase intake

Bulimia Nervosa

Summary: Normal or overweight patients who binge followed by a compensatory behavior
S/S: Eat an excessive amount of food rapidly, vomit/fast after, and feel remorse/guilt
Dx: Episodes occur at least 1 x week for 3 or more months; Russell's sign on PE
Treatment: CBT + SSRI mainstay of treatment

Pathophysiology:

- Primary hypothesis is a **serotonin imbalance**
  - Imbalance of pancreatic polypeptide YY which regulates pancreatic secretions and is responsible for satiety and slows gastric emptying - High PPYY means lower body weight from increased satiety and is "anorexigenic" - Sociocultural emphasis on being thin and participating in sports or activities that emphasize body size
- Binge episodes are usually triggered by stress
- Risk factors – adolescents (usually older than anorexia around age 20), **F>M**, genetics/culture

Clinical Manifestations:

- Episodes of binge eating followed by a compensatory behavior like purging, fasting, excessive exercise
- Binge - **Eating an excessive amount of food** (larger than most people would eat in the same amount of time) **rapidly with feelings of loss of control** (food is usually unhealthy and high in calories)
- Patients **feel guilty or remorseful** after their binge
- Patients may be **overweight or normal weight**
- Presenting signs may be gastritis/esophagitis secondary to acid exposure from repeated vomiting; parotitis (swollen parotid glands, can occur after cessation of vomiting behaviors)
- Physical exam – **Russell's sign** (abrasion/callus/scars on knuckles from self-induced vomiting), poor dentition
- Complications – Mallory Weiss/Boerhaave's, pancreatitis, swollen parotid glands

Diagnosis:

- DSM-5 – Binge eating + inappropriate compensatory behaviors both occur on average **at least once a week for ≥ 3 months:**
  - Recurrent episodes of binge eating, defined by: eating a larger portion of food than most people would eat in that same sitting AND lack of control over that eating
  - Recurrent compensatory behaviors to prevent gaining weight – inducing vomiting, misuse of laxatives/diuretics or other meds, fasting, or excessive exercise

- Additionally, self-evaluation is influenced by weight/body shape; and the above disturbances are not exclusively during episodes of anorexia nervosa

Treatment:

- **Combo of CBT + SSRI** + nutrition counseling is the best!
  - CBT – patients learn impulse control and change distorted thinking patterns
  - Fluoxetine (Prozac)/other SSRIs = mainstay
- AVOID bupropion (Wellbutrin) - contraindicated in eating disorders because it lowers seizure threshold (& seizure threshold is also lowered due to vomiting) and causes appetite suppression

Binge Eating Disorder

Summary: A lack of control → recurrent episodes of eating a large amount
S/S: Patients are overweight and have many complications from obesity
Dx: Sense of lack of control, overeating at least once/week ≥3 months + 3 BED sx
Tx: CBT is the best support tx, encourage weight loss and healthy lifestyle mods

Pathophysiology:
- Theories of pathophysiology
  - Decreased brain-derived neurotrophic factor (BDNF) - Helps to regulate eating behaviors - "maladaptation of the corticostriatal circuitry regulating motivation and impulse control"
  - Genetics
  - Low levels of serotonin (most studied)
- Risk factors – **M>F**, family hx, mood disorders, obesity (biggest), exposure to trauma, HTN

Clinical Manifestations:
- **Recurrent episodes of consuming a lot of food due to loss of control**, not followed by a compensatory behavior
- **Obesity, weight gain**
- Dry skin, GI issues, sleep problems
- Reluctance to discuss eating habits
- Metabolic syndrome – large waist, high triglycerides, low HDL, HTN, and high fasting blood glucose
- MSK complaints/chronic pain
- Mild to moderate depression

Diagnosis:
- DSM-5 – Patients have a sense of **lack of control overeating at least once a week for ≥3 months**:
  - An episode of binge eating is characterized by both of the following: Eating, in a discrete period of time an amount of food that is larger than what most people would eat AND a sense of lack of control overeating during the episode
  - The binge eating episodes are **associated ≥3 symptoms**:
    - Eating much more rapidly than normal
    - Eating until feeling uncomfortably full
    - Eating large amounts of food when not feeling physically hungry
    - Eating alone because of feeling embarrassed by how much one is eating, feeling disgusted with oneself, depressed, or very guilty afterward

- Marked distress regarding binge eating is present

- Not associated with the recurrent use of inappropriate compensatory behaviors

Treatment:

- **CBT** – most studied and best support treatment
- Encourage healthy lifestyle modifications - Weight loss, exercise, portion control
- Interpersonal psychotherapy
- SSRI may eliminate binge eating symptoms temporarily - Only use short term
- **Lisdexamfetamine (Vyvanse)** – only FDA approved med for BED
- Topiramate (Topamax) – suppresses appetite, but side effects
- GLP (semaglutide/tirzepitide) off label but sometimes used/helpful

Body Dysmorphic Disorder

Summary: Preoccupation of perceived flaws coupled with repetitive behaviors
S/S: mirror checking, excessive grooming/exercise w/ concerns to self-appearance
Dx: Preoccupation with a perceived flaw with repetitive coping behaviors
Tx: Cognitive-behavioral therapy, SSRIs

Pathophysiology:

- Theories of pathophysiology
  - Genetics – 8% have a family member with BDD and 7% have a family member with OCD
  - Low levels of serotonin
  - Preliminary research for proposed pathophysiology:
    - Association found between BDD and the gamma-aminobutyric acid (GABA)A-γ2 gene
    - BDD pts showed differences from controls in visual processing and abnormal amygdala activation, which could explain perceptual distortions
      - Tend to have a bias for analyzing visual specific details rather than the whole picture
    - MRI study found leftward shift in caudate volume asymmetry and greater total white matter volume (needs further study)
- Risk factors – childhood neglect and abuse, first-degree relative with OCD/body dysmorphic disorder (BDD), MC onset age 12-13, ⅔ of people onset prior to age 18
  - Associated with **high levels of anxiety**, social anxiety/avoidance, perfectionism, **depressed mood**, low extroversion, low self-esteem

Clinical Manifestations:

- **Negative perception of body coupled with compensatory behavior such as excessive grooming**
  - Obsessions and compulsions surrounding specifically physical attributes
  - Impaired psychosocial functioning (ex. avoidance of social outings)
- High rates of suicidal ideation and suicide attempts
- Can have comorbid OCD or eating disorder
- Muscle dysmorphia mostly in males

Diagnosis:

- DSM-5:

- A. Preoccupation with one or more perceived physical flaws which are slight/unnoticeable to others
- B. Perform repetitive behaviors at some point (excessive grooming, skin picking, reassurance seeking, repetitive mirror usage) or mental acts (comparing oneself to others)
- C. The preoccupation causes significant distress or social impairment in social, or other areas of functioning
- D. Not better explained by body concerns by someone whose symptoms meet criteria for an eating disorder

Treatment:

- CBT – most studied and best support treatment
- SSRI – first-line pharmacological treatment

SEXUAL RELATED DISORDERS

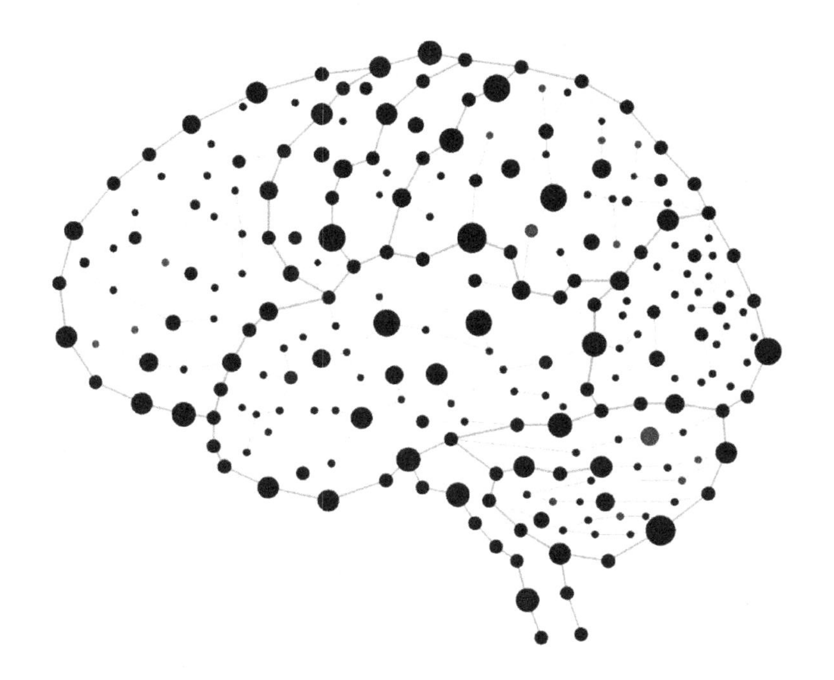

Exhibitionistic Disorder

Summary: A paraphilic disorder in which one finds pleasure revealing their genitals to strangers
S/S: Patients have a strong desire for others to watch their sexual acts
Dx: Criteria must be met for at least 6 months, and it must cause distress/impairment
Tx: Psychotherapy and medications (SSRI, leuprolide) are used

Pathophysiology:
- Many **sex offenders** have this disorder; onset during adolescence is common
- Risk factors – antisocial personality disorder, alcohol use disorder, pedophilia, sexual/emotional abuse, hypersexual
- Comorbidities are common – depressive, bipolar, anxiety, substance use disorder, hypersexuality, ADHD, antisocial personality disorder, other paraphilic disorders

Clinical Manifestations:
- Patients find **pleasure/excitement in revealing their genitals to an unsuspecting stranger**
- May have a strong desire for others to watch their sexual acts so they may become **adult entertainers**

Diagnosis:
- No minimum age requirement to diagnosis, so it is hard to differentiate if it is sexual curiosity
- DSM-5 – **over period of at least 6 months**, recurrent and intense **sexual arousal from exposure of one's genitals to an unsuspecting person,** as manifested by fantasies, urges, or behaviors. Individual has acted on sexual urges with a nonconsenting person, or sexual urges or fantasies cause clinically significant distress or impairment in social, occupational, or other important areas of functioning

Treatment:
- **Psychotherapy** – support groups are helpful
- Medications – **SSRI**; drugs to reduce testosterone (leuprolide or medroxyprogesterone)
- Can measure effectiveness of treatment using **penile plethysmography** (measures blood flow to penis with exposure to sexual stimuli)

Female Sexual Interest/Arousal Disorder

Summary: Lack of or reduced sexual desire preventing initiating sex or achieving orgasm
S/S: Absence/reduced sexual interest, thought, initiation of sex, excitement, and/or pleasure
Dx: ≥3 symptoms for ≥6 months causing distress and can't be explained medically
Tx: Varies – only FDA approved treatments are flibanserin, bremelanotide

Pathophysiology:

- Sexual dysfunction – A **problem during any phase of the sexual response cycle that prevents one from experiencing satisfaction** - More prevalent in women (35% of women >50 years old)
- Causes can be due to biological, psychological, or social factors
    - Illnesses/medications can lower androgen levels and lower sexual desire
    - Some medical conditions are associated with **painful intercourse such as endometriosis**
- Aging plays a role –
    - DHEA, which is associated with sexual desire, falls in the 30s and steadily decreases afterwards
    - Decreased estradiol occurs in menopause and leads to vaginal dryness, vaginal discomfort, and dyspareunia (result in loss of libido or intimacy avoidance)
- Risk factors – depression, anxiety, vascular disease, neurological conditions, gynecological issues (atrophy, lichen sclerosis, chronic infections), high stress, history of sexual abuse

Clinical Manifestations:

- The absence or reduced sexual interest, thoughts, initiation of sex, sexual excitement, sexual pleasure, sexual arousal, and/or genital/non-genital sensations during sex

Diagnosis:

- DSM-5 – Lack of or reduced sexual interest/arousal with **≥3 symptoms for ≥6 months**:
    - Absent/reduced interest in sexual activity
    - Absent/reduced sexual/erotic thoughts/fantasies
    - No/reduced initiation of sexual activity and unreceptive to partner's initiation
    - Absent/reduced sexual excitement/pleasure during sexual activity in almost all sexual encounters
    - Absent/reduced sexual interest in response to any internal/external sexual/erotic cues
    - Absent/reduced genital/non-genital sensations during sexual activity in most sexual encounters

- Symptoms cause distress and are not explained by a nonsexual mental disorder and are not attributable to a substance/medication or another medical condition
- Providers may opt to do a pelvic exam – check for vaginal atrophy, structural abnormality, pelvic tenderness, pelvic prolapse etc.
- Note – androgen levels are not tested since the assay test is not reliable and it isn't an independent predictor of low sex drive in women

Treatment:

- FDA approved medications
    - **Flibanserin (Addyi)** – treats low sexual desire in premenopausal women; works within 8 weeks; AE include hypotension, fatigue, nausea, dizziness, fainting
    - **Bremelanotide (Vyleesi)** – injection given before sexual activity that helps increase sex drive; AE include vomiting, flushing, headache, skin reaction
- Non-FDA approved medications:
    - Bupropion – may increase sexual responsiveness in females
    - **Testosterone** therapy (transdermal patch) has been shown to increase sexual desire in postmenopausal women or women menopausal from bilateral oophorectomies
- Management of vaginal dryness:
    - Topical lubricants and moisturizers can be used during sexual activity
    - Postmenopausal women – **low dose estrogen** (systemic or local) for vaginal dryness and atrophy
    - Dermal patch, vaginal ring, cream, pills
- **Cognitive behavioral therapy** and sex therapy

Male Hypoactive Sexual Desire Disorder

Summary: Many etiologies, though aging is the most common cause
S/S: Low desire, delay, infrequency, or absence of orgasm during sexual activity
Dx: ≥6-month absence or deficiency of sexual thoughts, desires, or fantasies causing distress
Tx: Psychological etiology – CBT w/behavior sex therapy; for hypogonadism – testosterone

Pathophysiology:

- Aging is the MC cause – **Men have a decline in testosterone in their 50s and in DHEA in their 30s**
- Other etiologies include illness, medications, psychological, biological, or social factors
- Risk factors – highest rate in older men and young men that are non-white, separated, less educated, and low income

Clinical Manifestations:

- **Low sexual desire, delay, infrequency, or absence of orgasm during sexual activity**
- Some have a lot of intercourse to please their significant other, therefore high frequency of sex does not rule out hypoactive disorder
- Men who ejaculate within one minute of sexual activity
- Specify onset and triggers
  - Lifelong disturbance – Present since individual became sexually active
  - Acquired disturbance – Began after a period of relatively normal sexual function
  - Generalized – Not limited to certain types of stimulation, situations, or partners
  - Situational – Only occurs with certain types of stimulation, situations, partners

Diagnosis:

- DSM-5 – Absence/deficiency of sexual thoughts, desire, or fantasies **for ≥6 months**:
  - May also have erectile dysfunction or abnormal ejaculation
  - May even engage in sex without desire in order to keep the relationship stable
  - Persistent, recurrent deficiency or absent sexual/erotic thoughts/fantasies for sexual activity
  - Symptoms cause clinically significant distress in the individual
  - Not attributable to the effects of a substance/medication or another medical condition

- Check for hair pattern, small testes, gynecomastia, pulses, visual loss due to pituitary tumor
- Test thyroid and prolactin levels for hypothyroidism or hyperprolactinemia
- **Low testosterone** – **Hypogonadism**

Treatment:

- Psychological etiology – **CBT with behavioral sex therapy**
- Low testosterone/hypogonadism – testosterone (cream, gel, patch, IM)
- If the cause is related to erectile dysfunction or premature ejaculation – treat underlying cause

Erectile Dysfunction (ED)

Summary: Inability to attain or sustain an erection secondary to organic or psychogenic cause
S/S: Psychogenic- Can have morning erection and ED is sudden onset and situational
Dx: ≥1 of the ED symptoms during most or all occasions of sexual act for ≥6 mo
Tx: Psychotherapy; PDE5 inhibitors 1st line (sildenafil/Viagra)

Pathophysiology:

- **Prevalence of ED is very high among men aged 40-70 (>50%)**
- Etiology
    - Primary – Male that has never been able to attain or sustain an erection
    - Secondary – Male that previously could attain/sustain an erection and later acquired ED
- Risk factors – aging (MC), systemic diseases (HTN, DM, HLD), endocrine disorders, alcohol abuse, smoking, trauma to pelvis/spine, stress, depression, medications (antihypertensives, antidepressants)

Clinical Manifestations:

- **Inability to obtain or sustain an erection for sexual intercourse**
- Psychogenic cause – Sudden onset and is usually situational
    - Ask about **morning erections** (typically will have a morning erection which rules out an organic etiology)
- Organic cause – Gradual onset, **occurs in all situations**
    - Men will not have morning erections
- Symptoms may cause low self-esteem, low self-confidence, decreased sense of masculinity, depression
- Men may **avoid sexual encounters** for fear of inability to perform
- Decreased sexual satisfaction/reduced desire in the individual's partner are common

Diagnosis:

- DSM-5 – **≥1 of the following symptoms during most or all occasions of sexual activity for ≥6 months**:
    - Marked difficulty in obtaining an erection during sexual activity
    - Marked difficulty in maintaining an erection through completion of activity
    - Marked decrease in erectile rigidity
- Symptoms cause clinically significant distress and not better explained by another disorder/medications
- Testing
    - **Nocturnal penile tumescence testing** and **measured erectile turgidity during sleep** will help differentiate

organic vs psychogenic erectile problems on the assumption that adequate erections during REM sleep indicate a psychological etiology to ED

- Doppler ultrasound, intravascular injection of vasoactive drugs, and other invasive diagnostic procedures can be used to assess vascular integrity
- Pudendal nerve conduction studies can be employed when peripheral neuropathy is suspected
- Decreased sexual desire in the patient warrants checking **free testosterone and thyroid function**
- Assess serum lipids if there is an increased risk of CAD in men ≥40 years old

Treatment:

- Psychotherapy for anxiety, depression, stress
- Sexual behavioral therapy and/or couples therapy for psychological causes
- Consider stopping medications which may be the cause of ED (especially antidepressants)
- Medications
  - **PDE5 Inhibitors** – inhibit phosphodiesterase
    - **Sildenafil (Viagra)**, vardenafil, avanafil, tadalafil
      - Contraindicated for those on nitrate therapy
  - Prostaglandin E1 analogue – alprostadil
    - Injected into the corpora cavernosa or transurethral and acts locally to produce an erection within 2-3 minutes, works in the absence of sexual stimulation

Fetishistic Disorder

Summary: Using a fetish to become sexually aroused
S/S: Steal or collect fetishes (shoes, leather, etc.); sexual dysfunction w/o the fetish
Dx: ≥6 months of sexual arousal from using a fetish on a body part that causes distress
Tx: Psychotherapy and SSRIs are used but have had limited success

Pathophysiology:

- Usually, individuals have more than one fetish that can be related (socks, shoes, feet) or unrelated
- **Onset is usually in puberty**, but fetish can develop before adolescence
- Comorbidities – other paraphilic disorders, hypersexuality, neurological conditions

Clinical Manifestations:

- **Using a fetish (inanimate object) to become sexually aroused and orgasm**
    - Fetish is used to describe sexual interests, preference for physical characteristics, preferred sexual activities but this disorder refers to the meaning of an inanimate object
- **Sexual dysfunction when fetish object or body part is unavailable** May prefer solitary sexual activity associated w/ fetish or incorporate the fetish into sexual activity
- May steal or collect fetishistic objects – aprons, shoes, leather, latex, **women's undergarments,** etc.
- Specify whether the patient has a fetish with body parts, nonliving objects, etc.

Diagnosis:

- DSM-5 – **For at least 6 months**, recurrent and intense sexual arousal from use of nonliving objects or a highly specific focus on congenital body part(s), as manifested by fantasies, urges, or behaviors. This causes clinically significant distress or impairment in social or occupational functioning
    - Fetish objects not limited to articles of clothing used in cross-dressing (transvestism) or devices specifically designed for the purpose of tactile genital stimulation (i.e. vibrator)

Treatment:

- Psychotherapy and SSRIs are used but have had limited success

Pedophile Disorder

Summary: Recurrent, sexually arousing fantasies/behaviors involving the prepubescent
S/S: Engages in/obsesses over sexual activity w/ children who are usually <13 y/o
Dx: ≥6 months, the individual is ≥ 16 years old and ≥5 years older than child
Tx: Psychotherapy; 1st line IM Medroxyprogesterone acetate to reduce testosterone and libido

Pathophysiology:
- MC a **family member or authority figure** (teacher, coach) versus it being a stranger
- Risk Factors – **sexual abuse**, neurodevelopmental disturbance in utero, M>F, interest in child pornography
- Comorbidities – substance use disorder, depression, bipolar, anxiety, antisocial personality disorder

Clinical Manifestations:
- **Recurrent, intense sexually arousing fantasies, sexual urges, or behaviors involving sexual activity with a prepubescent child or children**
  - Hebephilia – interest in children 11–14 and showing tanner stages 2 to 3 of physical development
  - Ephebophilia interest in late-pubescent youths in Tanner Stage 4 (ages 15-19)
- Individual has acted on sexual urges, or sexual urges or fantasies cause marked distress
- Does not include an individual in late adolescence involved in an ongoing sexual relationship (such as a 19-year-old dating a 16-year-old – illegal but does not meet criteria for pedophile disorder)
- **Types**
  - Exclusive type -Attracted only to children
  - Nonexclusive type - Attracted to adults as well as children
  - Limited to incest - Only attracted to children who are related to them

Diagnosis:
- DSM-5 – Period of at least **6 months, the individual is ≥ 16 years old and ≥5 years older than child**
  - Recurrent, intense sexually arousing fantasies or behaviors involving a child (usually ≤13 years old)
  - Has acted on urges or is greatly distressed/impaired by the urges (patients not always distressed)

Treatment:
- **Psychotherapy** (individual or group) – social skills training

- Treat any comorbidities – addition of an SSRI may be helpful
- Treatment of choice – **IM Medroxyprogesterone acetate** (blocks LH and FSH production from the pituitary to reduce testosterone which in turn, decreases libido)
- **Leuprolide** (GnRH agonist) which also reduces LH/FSH is 2nd line and requires less frequent injections
- Maintain testosterone levels in males in the normal female range (<62 ng/dL)

Sexual Masochism Disorder

Summary: Patients find pleasure in being humiliated (bound, beaten, abused, etc.)
S/S: Pt may find a sadist to humiliate them/inflict harm to live out sexual fantasies
Dx: ≥6 months of intense sexual arousal from humiliation and causes distress
Tx: There is currently no known effective treatment but psychotherapy can be tried

Pathophysiology:
- Comorbidities include other paraphilic disorders like transvestic fetishism
- Onset is usually in late teens and early 20s although can begin earlier on

Clinical Manifestations:
- **Intentional participation in a humiliating activity that involves being beaten, bound, or abused for pleasure that causes distress or impairs function**
- **Asphyxiophilia** – reduced oxygen to brain (by strangulation, suffocation, etc. enhances sexual arousal)
  - At increased risk of death and brain damage
- May act on masochistic fantasies on themselves – binding themselves, piercing their skin, burning oneself, shocking oneself
- May seek a sexual sadist so the partner can blindfold, whip, urinate/defecate on, bind them
- Patient may admit to watching pornography involving act of being humiliated, beaten, bound or suffering

Diagnosis:
- DSM-5 – **Over period of at least 6 months**, patients have recurrent and intense sexual arousal from act of being humiliated, beaten, bound, or suffering, as manifested by fantasies, urges, or behaviors
- Cause clinically significant **distress/impairment** in social and/or occupational functioning

Treatment:
- There is currently no known effective treatment but psychotherapy can be tried

Sexual Sadism Disorder

Summary: Patients who get pleasure from inflicting pain/suffering on others
S/S Engages in or obsesses over acts that inflict pain/suffering for pleasure
Dx: ≥6 months w/ intense sexual arousal from the suffering of another, non-consenting person
Tx: There is currently no known effective treatment but psychotherapy can be tried

Pathophysiology:

- Onset usually around age 19
- Majority of people practice sadistic behaviors, but the behavior doesn't meet diagnostic criteria
  - **Mild sadism between consenting adults is common**

Clinical Manifestations:

- A type of **paraphilia in which patients enjoy inflicting pain and suffering on a <u>non-consenting</u> adult**
- View pornography involved in the infliction of pain/suffering for pleasure

Remember:
Masochists hurt **me**
Sadists hurt **someone** else

Diagnosis:

- DSM-5 – **≥6 months with recurrent, intense sexual arousal from the suffering of another person**
  - Individual has acted on the urges with a nonconsenting person, or they cause impairment

Treatment:

- There is currently no known effective treatment but psychotherapy can be tried

Voyeuristic Disorder

Summary: Sexual arousal by observing a non-consenting person naked or engaging in sexual acts
S/S: Achieve pleasure during or after watching the act
Dx: Patient must be ≥18 years old, have ≥6 months of arousal from voyeurism, must cause distress
Tx: Psychotherapy and medications (SSRIs, leuprolide) are often used

Pathophysiology:
- MC disorder to result in **arrests** because getting caught is common
- Onset occurs in adolescence, usually around age 18 (<18 may be sexual curiosity)
- Risk factors – childhood sexual abuse, substance misuse, hypersexuality
- Comorbidities – hypersexuality, exhibitionistic disorder, depressive, bipolar, anxiety, substance use disorder, ADHD, conduct disorder, antisocial personality disorder

Clinical Manifestations:
- Sexual arousal by **observing a non-consenting person who is naked, undressing, or engaging in sexual activity.** May lead to problems with the law and with relationships
- Many with this disorder will **achieve pleasure during or after the activity** on their own via masturbation but do not usually seek sexual contact with the person they are observing
- Watching pornography is not considered voyeurism because it lacks the element of secret observation

Diagnosis:
- DSM-5 – **≥ 6 months** of recurrent and intense sexual arousal from observing unsuspecting person who is naked, disrobing, or engaging in sexual activity, as manifested by fantasies, urges, or behaviors
- Patient must be **≥ 18 years old**
- Individual has acted on sexual urges with nonconsenting person, or sexual urges/fantasies cause clinically significant impairment in social or occupational functioning

Treatment:
- **Psychotherapy** – support groups are helpful
- Medications – **SSRI,** drugs to reduce testosterone (leuprolide or medroxyprogesterone)

Frotteuristic Disorder

Summary: Paraphilia where pt is aroused by rubbing up on an unwilling person
S/Ss: Daydream about touching another person but has anxiety over their actions
Dx: Touching a non-consenting person at ≥3 times; behavior causes impairment for ≥6 months
Treatment: Psychotherapy

Pathophysiology:

- MC in males aged 15-25 years old
- Risk factors – antisocial behavior, hypersexuality
- Comorbidities – hypersexuality, paraphilic disorders, conduct, antisocial personality disorder, depressive, bipolar, anxiety, substance use disorders

Clinical Manifestations:

- Individuals are aroused by rubbing up against or touching another person
- Often occurs in crowded places where a person can easily escape like a subway or busy sidewalk
- May daydream about touching another person but also has anxiety from their actions

Diagnosis:

- DSM-5 – Recurrent and intense sexual arousal from touching or rubbing against a nonconsenting person, as manifested by fantasies, urges, or behaviors for ≥6 months. Individual has acted on sexual urges (minimum of 3 times) with a nonconsenting person, or the sexual urges or fantasies cause clinically significant distress or impairment in social or occupational function

Treatment:

- Psychotherapy – focuses on lessening the person's sexual desires and helps patients cope in healthy ways

ABBREVIATION KEY

Abbreviation	Explanation
A/C	Anticoagulation
A/w	Associated with
AA	African American
ADD	Attention Deficit Disorder
ADHD	Attention-Deficit / Hyperactivity Disorder
AE	Adverse Effects
AMS	Altered Mental Status
AODL	Activities of Daily Living
AOR	Assembly of Representatives
APAP	Acetaminophen/Tylenol
Asx	Asymptomatic
AUD	Alcohol Use Disorder
BAC	Blood Alcohol Concentration
BB	Beta Blocker
BED	Binge Eating Disorder
BG	Blood Glucose
BID	Twice a day
BP	Blood Pressure
Ca	Calcium
CBC	Complete Blood Count
CBT	Cognitive Behavioral Therapy
CCB	Calcium Channel Blocker
CI	Contraindicated
D/c	Discontinue
DA	Dopamine
DAPT	Dual Antiplatelet Therapy
DBT	Dialectical Behavior Therapy
DM	Diabetes Mellitus
DSM-5	Diagnostic Statistical Manual of Mental Disorders, 5th Ed
Dysfx	Disfunction
Dx	Diagnosis
ECT	Electro-Convulsive Therapy
EKG	Electrocardiogram

EPS	Extrapyramidal Symptoms
ER	Extended Release
ESR	Erythrocyte Sedimentation Rate
ETOH	Alcohol
F	Female
F/u	Follow-Up
Fe	Iron
FHx	Family History
FT4	Free T4
GAD	Generalized Anxiety Disorder
H/a	Headache
H/o	History of
H&H	Hemoglobin and Hematocrit
H2	Hydrogen
HA1c	Hemoglobin A1c
Hct	Hematocrit
Hgb	Hemoglobin
HLD	Hyperlipidemia
HPT	Hyperparathyroidism
HTN	Hypertension
Hx	History
IR	Immediate Release
IVDU	Intravenous Drug Use
IVF	In Vitro Fertilization
IVIG	Intravenous Immunoglobulin
K	Potassium
KOH	Potassium Hydroxide
LDL	Low-Density Lipoprotein
LFT	Liver Function Tests
MAOI	Monoamine Oxidase Inhibitors
MC (M/C)	Most Common
MCC (M/C/C)	Most Common Cause
MDD	Major Depressive Disorder
MOA	Mechanism of Action
MSM	Gay, bisexual, and other men who have sex with men
N/V/D/C	Nausea/Vomiting/Diarrhea/Constipation
Na	Sodium

NAC	N-Acetylcysteine
NDRI	Norepinephrine and Dopamine Reuptake Inhibitors
NE	Norepinephrine
NMDA	N-Methyl-D-Aspartate
NRI	Norepinephrine Reuptake Inhibitors
OCD	Obsessive Compulsive Disorder
OD	Overdose
OTC	Over the Counter
Patho	Pathophysiology
PHQ	Patient Health Questionnaire
PMDD	Premenstrual Dysphoric Disorder
PMH	Past Medical History
PMS	Premenstrual Syndrome
PRL	Prolactin
PRN	As Needed
Pts	Patients
PTSD	Post-Traumatic Stress Disorder
R/O	Rule Out
RF	Risk Factor(s)
Tx	Treatment
S/S	Signs/Symptoms
SA	Serotonin
SAD	Seasonal Affective Disorder
SNS	Sympathetic Nervous System
SSRI	Selective Serotonin Reuptake Inhibitors
SX	Symtoms
TBI	Traumatic Brain Injury
TCA	Tricyclic Antidepressants
TFTs	Thyroid Function Tests
TSH	Thyroid Stimulating Hormone
Tx	Treatment
W/	With
W/in	Within
W/O	Without
WBC	White Blood Cell(s)
y/o	Years Old

References

"Adderall vs. Vyvanse: What's the Difference?" *American Addiction Centers*, 23 Feb. 2021, americanaddictioncenters.org/adderall/vs-vyvanse.

"Alcohol Withdrawal." *Harvard Health*, www.health.harvard.edu/a_to_z/alcohol-withdrawal-a-to-z.

Attia, Evelyn, and B. Timothy Walsh. "Psychiatric Disorders." *Merck Manuals Professional Edition*, Merck Manuals, www.merckmanuals.com/professional/psychiatric-disorders/eating-disorders/bulimia-nervosa?query=bulimia.

Barnhill, John W. "Psychiatric Disorders." *Merck Manuals Professional Edition*, Merck Manuals, www.merckmanuals.com/professional/psychiatric-disorders/anxiety-and-stressor-related-disorders/adjustment-disorders?query=adjustment+disorder.

Berman, Brian D. "Neuroleptic Malignant Syndrome: a Review for Neurohospitalists." *The Neurohospitalist*, SAGE Publications, Jan. 2011, www.ncbi.nlm.nih.gov/pmc/articles/PMC3726098/#:~:text=In%20more%20severe%20cases%20of,release%20from%20the%20sarcoplasmic%20reticulum.

Brown, George R. "Psychiatric Disorders." *Merck Manuals Professional Edition*, Merck Manuals, www.merckmanuals.com/professional/psychiatric-disorders/sexuality,-gender-dysphoria,-and-paraphilias/exhibitionistic-disorder?redirectid=38&query=exhibitionistic+behaviors.

Brown, Kristin W., and Tyler J. Armstrong. "Hydrocarbon inhalation." *StatPearls*. StatPearls Publishing, 18 July 2022, www.ncbi.nlm.nih.gov/books/NBK470289.

Coryell, William. "Psychiatric Disorders." *Merck Manuals Professional Edition*, Merck Manuals, www.merckmanuals.com/professional/psychiatric-disorders/mood-disorders/bipolar-disorders?query=bipolar+disorder.

"Deep Brain Stimulation." *Mayo Clinic*, Mayo Foundation for Medical Education and Research, 7 Aug. 2020, www.mayoclinic.org/tests-procedures/deep-brain-stimulation/about/pac-20384562.

Diagnostic and Statistical Manual of Mental Disorders: DSM-5. American Psychiatric Association, 2017.

Dimsdale, Joel E. "Somatic Symptom Disorder - Psychiatric Disorders." *Merck Manuals Professional Edition*, Merck Manuals, www.merckmanuals.com/professional/psychiatric-disorders/somatic-symptom-and-related-disorders/somatic-symptom-disorder?query=somatic+symptom+disorder.

Elia, Josephine. "Oppositional Defiant Disorder (ODD) - Pediatrics." *Merck Manuals Professional Edition*, Merck Manuals, www.merckmanuals.com/professional/pediatrics/mental-disorders-in-children-and-adolescents/oppositional-defiant-disorder-odd?query=oppositional+defiant+disorder.

"Female Sexual Dysfunction." *Mayo Clinic*, Mayo Foundation for Medical Education and Research, 17 Dec. 2020, www.mayoclinic.org/diseases-conditions/female-sexual-dysfunction/diagnosis-treatment/drc-20372556.

Feusner, Jamie D., Jose Yaryura-Tobias, and Sanjaya Saxena. "The pathophysiology of body dysmorphic disorder." *Body Image* 5.1, March 2008, https://www.ncbi.nlm.nih.gov/pmc/articles/PMC3836287.

First, Michael B. "Behavioral Emergencies - Psychiatric Disorders." *Merck Manuals Professional Edition*, Merck Manuals, Feb. 2020, www.merckmanuals.com/professional/psychiatric-disorders/approach-to-the-patient-with-mental-symptoms/behavioral-emergencies?query=homicide.

"First-Generation Antipsychotics ." *UpToDate*, www.uptodate.com/contents/first-generation-antipsychotic-medications-pharmacology-administration-and-comparative-side-effects#H272233927.

"Generalized Anxiety Disorder 7-Item (GAD-7)." *National HIV Curriculum*, www.hiv.uw.edu/page/mental-health-screening/gad-7.

Greenblatt, Karl, and Ninos Adams. "Modafinil." *StatPearls*. StatPearls Publishing, 6 Feb. 2023, https://www.ncbi.nlm.nih.gov/books/NBK531476.

Gupta, Rishab. "Pralidoxime." *NCBI*, 12 July 2022, https://www.ncbi.nlm.nih.gov/books/NBK558908.

"Helpful for Chronic Pain in Addition to Depression." *Mayo Clinic*, Mayo Foundation for Medical Education and Research, 5 Oct. 2019, www.mayoclinic.org/diseases-conditions/depression/in-depth/antidepressants/art-20044970.

Hirsch, Irvin H. "Erectile Dysfunction - Genitourinary Disorders." *Merck Manuals Professional Edition*, Merck Manuals, www.merckmanuals.com/professional/genitourinary-disorders/male-sexual-dysfunction/erectile-dysfunction?query=erectile+dysfunction.

"Insomnia." *Mayo Clinic*, Mayo Foundation for Medical Education and Research, 15 Oct. 2016, www.mayoclinic.org/diseases-conditions/insomnia/diagnosis-treatment/drc-20355173.

KM, Lenora. "Frotteuristic Disorder: Causes, Symptoms, Treatment DSM-5 302.89 (F65.81) ." *Thriveworks*, 15 Feb. 2018, thriveworks.com/blog/frotteuristic-disorder.

Lautieri, Amanda. "How Long Do Opiates Stay in Your System: Oxycodone & Hydrocodone." *American Addiction Centers*, 20 Oct. 2020, americanaddictioncenters.org/prescription-drugs/how-long-in-system.

Lewis, Cassaundra B., and Ninos Adams. "Phenobarbital." *StatPearls*. StatPearls Publishing, 17 Jan. 2022, https://www.ncbi.nlm.nih.gov/books/NBK532277.

"Male Hypoactive Sexual Disorder." *Serin Center*, 7 Dec. 2020, serincenter.com/treatments/male-hypoactive-sexual-disorder.

Mamo DC;Sweet RA;Keshavan. "Managing Antipsychotic-Induced Parkinsonism." *Drug Safety*, U.S. National Library of Medicine, pubmed.ncbi.nlm.nih.gov/10221855/#:~:text=Several%20strategies%20are%20utilised%20in,as%20anticholinergic%20agents%20and%20amantadine.

Mehanna, Hisham M, et al. "Refeeding Syndrome: What It Is, and How to Prevent and Treat It." *BMJ (Clinical Research Ed.)*, BMJ Publishing Group Ltd., 28 June 2008, www.ncbi.nlm.nih.gov/pmc/articles/PMC2440847.

Memon MD, Mohammed. "Panic Disorder." *Background, Etiology, Epidemiology*, Medscape, 6 Dec. 2020, emedicine.medscape.com/article/287913-overview.

"Narcolepsy." *Mayo Clinic*, Mayo Foundation for Medical Education and Research, 6 Nov. 2020, www.mayoclinic.org/diseases-conditions/narcolepsy/diagnosis-treatment/drc-20375503.

Overview of Personality Disorders By Andrew Skodol, and Andrew Skodol. "Overview of Personality Disorders - Psychiatric Disorders." *Merck Manuals Professional Edition*, Merck Manuals, www.merckmanuals.com/professional/psychiatric-disorders/personality-disorders/overview-of-personality-disorders?query=personality+disorders.

O'Malley, Gerald F., and Rika O'Malley. "Injuries; Poisoning." *Merck Manuals Professional Edition*, Merck Manuals, www.merckmanuals.com/professional/injuries-poisoning/poisoning/acetaminophen-poisoning?query=acetaminophen.

Phillips, Katharine A., and Dan J. Stein. "Obsessive-Compulsive Disorder (OCD) - Psychiatric Disorders." *Merck Manuals Professional Edition*, Merck Manuals, Jan. 2021, www.merckmanuals.com/professional/psychiatric-disorders/obsessive-compulsive-and-related-disorders/obsessive-compulsive-disorder-ocd?query=obsessive+compulsive+disorder.

Prochaska, Judith J. "Smoking Cessation - Special Subjects." *Merck Manuals Professional Edition*, Merck Manuals, www.merckmanuals.com/professional/special-subjects/tobacco-use/smoking-cessation#v8545269.

Rahman, Masum. "Valproic Acid." *StatPearls* , U.S. National Library of Medicine, 26 Jan. 2021, www.ncbi.nlm.nih.gov/books/NBK559112/#:~:text=Go%20to%3A-,Mechanism%20of%20Action,also%20by%20inhibiting%20histone%20deacetylase.

Ricciardi, Lucia, et al. "Treatment Recommendations for Tardive Dyskinesia." *Canadian Journal of Psychiatry. Revue Canadienne De Psychiatrie*, SAGE Publications, June 2019, www.ncbi.nlm.nih.gov/pmc/articles/PMC6591749.

The Royal Children's Hospital Melbourne, www.rch.org.au/clinicalguide/guideline_index/Anticholinergic_Syndrome/#:~:text=Anticholinergic%20syndrome%20results%20from%20competitive,objects%20%2D%20which%20characterises%20this%20toxidrome.

"Sexual Disorder Symptoms – Sexual Masochism and Sadism." *Mental Help Sexual Disorder Symptoms Sexual Masochism and Sadism Comments*, www.mentalhelp.net/sexual-disorders/sexual-masochism-and-sadism/#:~:text=Sexual%20Masochism%3A,or%20otherwise%20made%20to%20suffer.

"Sexual Disorder Symptoms – Voyeurism." *Mental Help Sexual Disorder Symptoms Voyeurism Comments*, www.mentalhelp.net/sexual-disorders/voyeurism.

Soreff, MD, Stephen. "Attention Deficit Hyperactivity Disorder (ADHD)." *Background, Pathophysiology, Epidemiology*, Medscape, 26 Mar. 2020, emedicine.medscape.com/article/289350-overview#a6.

Spiegel, David. "Psychiatric Disorders." *Merck Manuals Professional Edition*, Merck Manuals, www.merckmanuals.com/professional/psychiatric-disorders/dissociative-disorders/depersonalization-derealization-disorder.

Spiegel, David. "Dissociative Amnesia - Psychiatric Disorders." *Merck Manuals Professional Edition*, Merck

"Table 3.32, DSM-IV to DSM-5 Illness Anxiety Disorder Comparison - Impact of the DSM-IV to DSM-5 Changes on the National Survey on Drug Use and Health - NCBI Bookshelf." *Impact of the DSM-IV to DSM-5 Changes on the National Survey on Drug Use and Health [Internet].*, U.S. National Library of Medicine, www.ncbi.nlm.nih.gov/books/NBK519704/table/ch3.t32/.

"Transcranial Magnetic Stimulation." *Mayo Clinic*, Mayo Foundation for Medical Education and Research, 27 Nov. 2018, www.mayoclinic.org/tests-procedures/transcranial-magnetic-stimulation/about/pac-20384625.

"Vagus Nerve Stimulation." *Mayo Clinic*, Mayo Foundation for Medical Education and Research, 17 Nov. 2020, www.mayoclinic.org/tests-procedures/vagus-nerve-stimulation/about/pac-20384565.

Victorio, M. Cristina. "Tic Disorders and Tourette Syndrome in Children and Adolescents - Pediatrics." *Merck Manuals Professional Edition*, Merck Manuals, Oct. 2019, www.merckmanuals.com/professional/pediatrics/neurologic-disorders-in-children/tic-disorders-and-tourette-syndrome-in-children-and-adolescents?query=tourette+syndrome.

Wagener, Dan. "Norepinephrine and Dopamine Reuptake Inhibitors (NDRIs)." *American Addiction Centers*, 4 Sept. 2019, americanaddictioncenters.org/antidepressants-guide/ndris.

Warner, Christopher H., et al. "Antidepressant Discontinuation Syndrome." *American Family Physician*, 1 Aug. 2006, www.aafp.org/afp/2006/0801/p449.html.

"What Is Autism?" *Autism Speaks*, www.autismspeaks.org/what-autism.

INDEX

First Line Guide, began with the Complete Review of Didactic and Clinical Medicine (3rd edition pictured below) first published in 2022, and more commonly known as FLG.

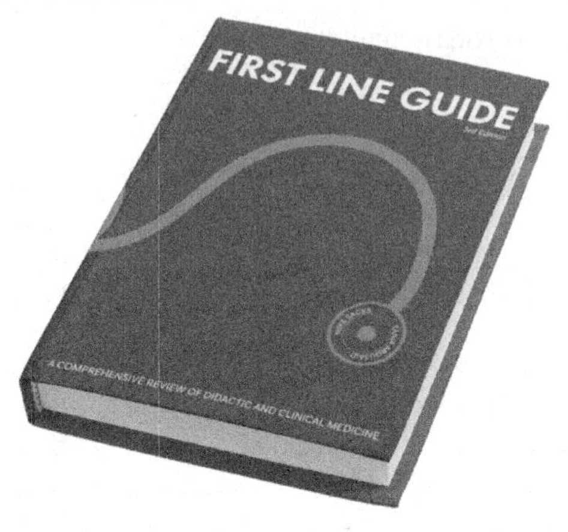

The first edition of FLG was written to fill many gaps that we saw in the market for both students of medicine, and those early in their clinical careers. Most importantly we set out to simplify the study of medicine, a topic we felt was almost purposely over-complicated.

In full color and more than 600 pages, FLG attempts to cover all topics of medicine using a body system approach and is an ideal study companion for students, and desk reference for general practitioners.

Based on the feedback of readers, and with the successes of the first two editions as a catalyst, in 2023 we set out to write smaller specialty focused editions for those on clinical clerkships and those entering/transitioning into specialties. This book, First Line Guide: Psychiatric and Behavioral Medicine, is the first in a series of these specialist focused books in production.

In early 2024, we published the 3rd edition, or FLG 3 to continued rave reviews as we've found a place as required reading in some programs of higher medical education.

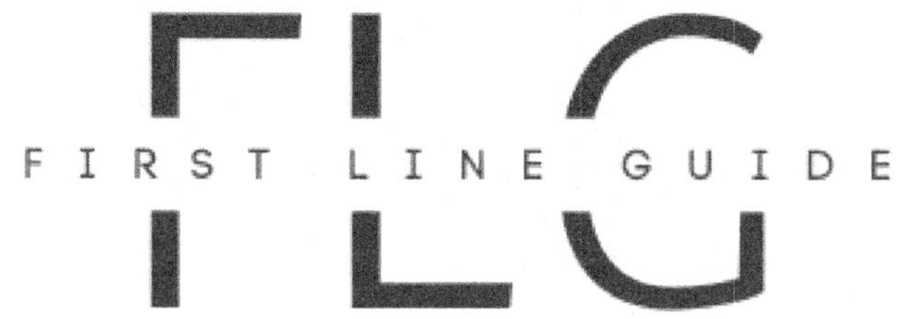

Made in the USA
Columbia, SC
25 July 2025